ROTATIONS

Also by Robert Marion, M.D.

Born Too Soon

The Intern Blues

The Boy Who Felt No Pain

Learning to Play God

Was George Washington Really the Father of Our Country?

ROTATIONS
The Twelve Months of Intern Life

Robert Marion, M.D.

HarperCollins*Publishers*

FIRST EDITION

Designed by Interrobang Design Studio

Library of Congress Cataloging-in-Publication Data

Marion, Robert.
    Rotations : the twelve months of intern life / by Robert Marion.
        p. cm.
    Includes index.
    ISBN 0-06-017263-0
    1. Interns (Medicine)—United States—Biography. 2. Interns (Medicine)—Job stress—United States.   I. Title.
  R123.M247   1997
   610'.71'55—dc21   97-4135

---

97 98 99 00 01 ❖/RRD 10 9 8 7 6 5 4 3 2 1

To my parents, Ann and Sam Marion, my mother-in-law, Mildred Schoenbrun, and to the memory of my father-in-law, Dr. Gerald Schoenbrun, who survived being on call every other night for one year

PROLOGUE

The Road to the First Rotation

This afternoon in my office, I saw Molly Richardson, a twelve-year-old girl referred to me for genetic evaluation. On a routine visit two weeks before, Molly's pediatrician had noticed that the girl had developed about a dozen darkly pigmented spots on the skin of her trunk. Knowing that these lesions—called café-au-lait spots, because they are the color of coffee with milk—could be a sign of a fairly common genetic disorder called neurofibromatosis, the pediatrician, who worked for one of the larger health maintenance organizations in New York, had put through the paperwork authorizing the visit.

The girl had always been in excellent health. Upon examining her, I found not only a total of sixteen café-au-lait spots on her skin, but also clusters of freckles in her armpits and a few small, rubbery lumps under the skin of her left arm—lumps I knew resulted from the enlargement of the cells that line peripheral nerves, a clear sign of neurofibromatosis.

After the exam was completed, I spent a few minutes explaining the features of the disease to Molly and her mother. I described the disorder's inheritance pattern; its recently discovered molecular, biochemical, and physiologic bases; and its generally favorable long-term prognosis. Near the end of the session, the girl's mother, not exactly overjoyed that I'd just confirmed her daughter had a potentially life-threatening condition, asked, "Well, Dr. Marion, where do we go from here?"

I answered that although most patients with neurofibromatosis spend their lives in excellent health, about one in ten develop some of the more serious consequences of the disorder, which can include brain tumors. I told her that because of this risk, it was important that Molly have some baseline tests, including an MRI (magnetic resonance imaging) of her head and spine, a careful ophthalmological exam, and a hearing test. Finally, I said that in order to try to pick up the known potential problems as early as possible, it was important that Molly have careful, regular follow-up and that some of these tests be repeated every six to twelve months for the rest of the girl's life.

The mother, considering this information for a few seconds, said, "Well, doctor, how soon can we get these tests done?"

That's when the trouble began.

In the old days (meaning prior to 1993), getting this workup done was a cinch: I'd simply pick up the phone and call our hospital's radiology department and schedule the MRIs; then I'd call ophthalmology to make arrangements for a visit to the pediatric eye doctor and ENT to schedule an audiogram. Having worked with people in these three departments for years, referring to them numerous patients with neurofibromatosis, I knew that the purpose of Molly's visits would be instantly understood. Finally, following completion of the evaluations, I'd schedule Molly to come back to my office for a follow-up visit, at which time I'd review with the family the results of the tests and discuss the plans for Molly's future medical needs.

But that's how things were done in the old days. Since the advent of managed care, life for medical specialists and their patients has become increasingly complicated. Not only am I now not permitted to schedule tests for patients where and when I want them done, but I have to first call the patient's primary care provider and plead my case about why these tests are medically necessary in the first place. Then, if I'm successful in my argument and manage to convince the primary care provider, I next have to find out where and when those visits will occur, call the people who will be performing the evaluations (specialists who, during the course of their careers, may never have had any experience with patients with neurofibromatosis), and explain to them exactly what it is that concerns me. Finally, I have to make sure the primary care provider will authorize a second visit to my office so that the results can be discussed and follow-up plans can be made.

This story about the roadblocks that got in the way of providing appropriate care for Molly may sound like nothing more than just another overtrained medical subspecialist spoiled by the easy life that existed prior to the advent of managed care. But this scenario has removed an important quality assurance from healthcare delivery: Molly's tests will be performed and interpreted not by people who are experts in neurofibromatosis, but by specialists who have simply signed a contract with the managed care company, providers who may have never seen a patient with this condition. Although the time wasted on arranging Molly's testing and follow-up may not seem like a big issue, when you multiply the minutes spent in making those phone calls and arguing with various members of the managed care organization's staff by the number of patients seen during the course of a week, you begin to understand the magnitude of the problem. The baggage that accompanies managed care has made providing excellent care to patients extremely difficult.

Undoubtedly, managed care has changed the way medicine

is practiced in the United States in the 1990s. And from the perspective of both a medical subspecialist and a patient, I don't believe these changes are in anyone's best interest—anyone, that is, except the HMO's officers and stockholders.

A revolution is occurring in American medicine. In the past five years, while managed care has spread like a cancer, what we knew as old-time private practice—the ability of a physician recently out of training to hang up a shingle, open an office, and just see patients—has died an ugly and undignified death. In medical schools and residency training programs throughout the country, the message that has come down from the federal government (the ultimate underwriter of those schools and programs) is that the overwhelming thrust of medical education should be focused on the training of family practitioners, generalists, internists, and pediatricians. Primary care is definitely in; subspecialty care is unquestionably out.

In New York City, the managed care revolution has changed the face of medicine in ways that none of us who work here would have ever dreamed possible. The revolution has brought about mergers between medical schools and teaching hospitals previously so independent, so chauvinistic, and so impressed with themselves that, five years ago, they would barely acknowledge one another's existence. These marriages and mergers have created gigantic medical monoliths, institutions trying to "corner the market" and gain monopolies in the delivery of care in various areas. Throughout the city, these developments have weakened and financially ruined many smaller, community-based facilities. Eventually, these changes will undoubtedly topple New York City's massive Health and

Hospitals Corporation, the largest municipal healthcare system in the world.

These staggering changes have not been confined to the administration of hospitals; there have been major alterations in the way we train young doctors as well. In July 1989, New York became the first state to institute laws regulating the working conditions of doctors-in-training. Prior to the adoption of these guidelines, which were recommended to the state's Department of Health by a commission headed by Dr. Bertrand Bell, a professor of internal medicine at the Albert Einstein College of Medicine in the Bronx, there were no regulations governing the training of house officers. Before 1989, interns and residents typically worked more than 110 hours per week, spending 36 or more hours in the hospital during a single on-call shift, and 24 or more hours in the emergency room without relief. The new regulations limited the number of hours an intern could work to 80 per week, with no more than 24 hours continuously as part of a single shift, and no more than 12 consecutive hours working in an ER.

I was an early and enthusiastic supporter of the work done by the Bell Commission. When the regulations went into effect, I believed they would cure a great number of ills inherent in the system we use to train young doctors. Having survived my own residency, having spent part of my professional career serving as an adviser to other house officers as they struggled through this archaic system of forced servitude, and having spent hours speaking with a large number of hospitalized patients, I knew that something needed to be done to reform this dangerous and unhealthy system. In 1989, I believed the new guidelines provided a first step, a start to a reform movement that would ultimately benefit not only the doctors-in-training, but that, more important, would improve the care given to patients hospitalized in America's large teaching hospitals.

I had good reason to hope the Bell Commission's recommendations would bring about such changes. I published *The Intern Blues: The Private Ordeals of Three Young Doctors*. The edited, transcribed diaries of three interns who were then training in the pediatric residency program at the medical school at which I work, the book paints a realistic picture of what training was like in the days just before the new regulations went into effect. In the final paragraph of the book, I concluded: "Everybody who lives through an internship is forever changed by the experience. The intern learns about the human body; he or she truly becomes a physician. But in the process, through the wearing down of the intern's spirit, that person also loses something he or she carried, some innocence, some humanness, some fundamental respect. The question is, Is it all worth it?"

More than seven years have now passed since the regulations first recommended by Dr. Bell's commission went into effect, enough time to evaluate their effect on all aspects of medicine. The question is, Has the institution of these guidelines created the revolution in residency training that I and others believed it would? The only way to answer this question with certainty is to reproduce the experiment of *The Intern Blues*, to follow, using tape-recorded diaries, three interns through their first year of training in the period after the new regulations went into effect and compare the experiences of *The Intern Blues* doctors with the more recently trained doctors. This experiment is the basis of this book.

On Thursday morning, June 23, 1994, I found myself once again sitting on the lawn outside the home of Peter Anderson, the chairman of the department of pediatrics at the Albert

Schweitzer School of Medicine. As had been the case nine long years before on the day when *The Intern Blues* began, I was surrounded by a group of people who, although looking well rested and well tanned, were unbelievably tightly wound. The occasion for this meeting of neurotic young doctors was our department's annual orientation retreat, and these people were the incoming class of interns.

During the course of that morning, the new interns expressed, virtually word for word, the same concerns raised during the retreat nine years before: They worried they hadn't learned enough in medical school and weren't technically competent to function as interns; they worried they would be overworked and that their lives outside of the hospital would suffer as a result; they worried that they wouldn't be able to handle the responsibilities that come with being a doctor.

It was during the introductory session that I announced my plan to replicate the situation of *The Intern Blues*. I told the group I would be enlisting the aid of three new interns who would be willing to keep tape-recorded diaries similar to those kept by Andy Baron, Mark Greenberg, and Amy Horowitz, the house officers whose experiences formed the basis of the earlier book. Happily, I found that not only did most of the interns know what I was talking about, but some actually seemed enthusiastic about participating in the project.

That morning, as I had done nine years earlier, I handed out tape recorders and blank tapes to six people. As was the case in 1985 and 1986, three members of that group of six faithfully made regular diary entries. It is the excerpts from the diaries of these three interns, who in the pages of this book are called Hal Burkins, Scott Lindsay, and Denise Powers, that form the study group whose experiences I will compare to those of Amy, Mark, and Andy.

•

Scientifically speaking, the only way to accurately measure the effects of the Bell Commission regulations on the lives of these interns is to keep all other variables exactly the same. As such, all other aspects of the trainees' lives in the hospital, including the working conditions, the wards on which they work, the rotation schedule, the patient population, and the members of the medical staff with whom they interact, should all remain unchanged. Unfortunately, since change has been such a prevalent part of medicine since the time of *The Intern Blues*, the internships experienced by Hal, Scott, and Denise were far from identical to those through which Andy, Mark, and Amy had labored and managed to survive.

For example, the federal government has put pressure on residency training programs to decrease the number of doctors being trained, and our program has clearly felt the effects of this pressure. Thirty-six new interns attended the orientation retreat at Peter Anderson's house in 1985; when the exercise was repeated in 1994, only twenty-four new doctors were sitting on the lawn.

This marked decrease in the number of trainees has brought with it a concurrent shrinkage in the number of locales in which house officers are required to work. When Andy Baron, Mark Greenberg, and Amy Horowitz began their training, pediatric interns in our program rotated through the services of four different hospitals: Mount Scopus, our main teaching hospital; University Hospital, a small, voluntary facility run by the administration of Mount Scopus located adjacent to our affiliated medical school; the Albert Schweitzer School of Medicine; and West Bronx Hospital and Jonas Bronck Medical Center, two municipal facilities run by New York City's Health and Hospitals Corporation. On the day Hal Burkins, Scott Lindsay, and Denise Powers began working, the number of hospitals had been cut from four to three. Interns are no longer assigned to the pediatric ward at University Hospital, and the experience at Jonas Bronck Medical Center had been substantially curtailed. Today, most interns spend only two months at the Bronck; others spend no time there at all.

Similarly, the number of inpatient services through which interns rotate has also been rolled back. Back in the days of *The Intern Blues*, first-year house officers were assigned to work on ten different wards, including two neonatal intensive care units. They worked in three emergency rooms and four separate clinic settings. Today, rotations occur on only six wards, including one NICU, two emergency rooms, and three clinics.

But although the setting for internship is somewhat more limited than in 1985, the experiences are otherwise comparable: The patient population is the same, the department's faculty is largely unchanged, and the professionals staffing the wards, emergency rooms, and clinics are similar. As such, the experiment should work.

Although all the events written about in this book are by and large true, some of the facts have been altered in order to provide the subjects with as much anonymity as possible. The names of the doctors, patients, staff members, hospitals, and medical schools have been changed for the same reason.

This book was the result of a group effort. I'd like to thank the interns who participated in this exercise, people who chose to devote some of the precious little free time they had to recording their impressions of life as house officers. Also, I'd like once again to thank the three interns whose lives were chronicled in *The Intern Blues*. Although they've spread themselves over the face of the Earth and gone on to pursue very different careers, I still am indebted to them for the assistance they provided way back when they were beginning their training.

Once again, I'd like to thank my friend and agent, Diana Finch, for always having time to answer some of the most ridiculous questions ever asked by a client. Also, thanks to Framji Minwalla at HarperCollins, who did a terrific and loving job editing the manuscript. And to Adrian Zackheim, my editor at HarperCollins, for his tremendous insight and literary acumen; Adrian, I don't know how you do it, but somehow, you always seem to be right!

Finally, I'd like to thank my children, Isadora, Davida, and Jonah, for allowing me the time to stare at the computer when I should have been out spending quality time with them; and once again, to Beth, who's shown amazing understanding during the good times and the bad times when this book was being written.

Robert Marion, M.D.
October 24, 1996

I

J U L Y

The First Rotation:
The Beginning of the End

Part 1: It's July 1; Whatever You Do, Don't Get Sick

> *My internship officially starts tomorrow. I've waited for this day*
> *a long time, years, the way people wait for their arteries to clog up*
> *enough for them to have a heart attack.*
> Mark Greenberg, June 28, 1985

In teaching hospitals throughout the United States, the evolutionary wheel of residency training completes its rotation on the first of July. On that day, senior residents—the people who just the day before literally ran the service—graduate from the grind of their training and leave to become attending physicians.

The liberation of these senior residents creates an immediate niche in the food chain. The seniors are replaced by junior residents; the suddenly vacant junior residency spots are immediately filled by former interns; and new doctors, people who only weeks before were carefree fourth-year medical students, become interns, doctors who, more than any other house officers, have direct responsibility for care of the patients.

The take-home message of this annual turning is: Whatever you do, don't get sick in the beginning of July!

Although they were separated by fifteen years, the start of my internship and the experiences shared by Hal Burkins, Scott Lindsay, and Denise Powers, the three interns whose lives I followed during 1994 and 1995, were not all that different. After my graduation on the first Tuesday of June 1979, my wife, Beth, and I packed our belongings, ready to vacate the apartment in the Bronx where we'd lived since getting married two years before.

Our move was going to be complicated. Beth, then a graduate student at Columbia University, was still working on her research; in order to allow her to finish her work, she had taken a dorm room on campus. Meanwhile, I was moving the bulk of our stuff to an apartment in Watertown, a suburb just west of Boston. Our plan was that Beth would spend weekdays in New York and come up to join me in Watertown on weekends.

But separating our possessions was not easy. For the better part of a week, Beth and I sorted and packed, argued and compromised, stopped speaking and made up, rarely got out, and certainly never had the opportunity to enjoy that beautiful spring. Finally, the job was complete. At eight o'clock on the morning of June 15, a United Van Lines truck came to move our stuff to Massachusetts. Our work, for the moment, was done, and it was time to do some celebrating.

Or maybe not. During the spring and summer of 1979, the Arab oil embargo was at its peak. Getting gas for cars was difficult, but keeping a fleet of moving vans on the road was apparently near impossible. Although our contract stipulated that the moving company would deliver our stuff within a week of pickup, the oil embargo made that contract moot. United Van Lines promised they'd get our belongings to Watertown as soon as possible—this turned out to be the end of August. In the meantime, I was told to make do as best as I could.

So I spent the night prior to my first day of internship (and too many nights thereafter) sleeping—or, more accurately, trying to sleep—in a sleeping bag on the floor of our empty apartment. But even if I'd been in my own bed, I'm pretty sure I wouldn't have gotten any sleep that night. All that evening, I'd been gripped by a strange mix of emotions that made relaxation nearly impossible: I was excited about finally beginning something I'd worked toward all my life, yet tense and scared that I wouldn't be good enough, that I wasn't well prepared, that I didn't know enough to be a good doctor. With all this swirling through my head, a queasiness in my stomach, and my hands and feet cold and clammy, I lay in my sleeping bag trying my best to fall asleep. I failed miserably.

The next morning as I approached the hospital, I felt these symptoms crescendo. My hands actually shook as I held the steering wheel of my car. A few times during the trip, I thought for sure I was going to vomit. To keep the nausea under control, I took deep breaths.

Finally, I was there. Even now, more than fifteen years later, I remember my last few seconds of freedom: As I approached the hospital's front door, I said a silent prayer asking God to help me get through this. Then I took one last deep breath of fresh air. I wanted to hold off breathing hospital air for as long as I could. I walked through the doors of the hospital holding my breath, heading toward the elevator.

I started my internship at St. Ann's, a women's and babies' hospital in South Boston affiliated with Boston Medical Center, the main teaching hospital at which I'd be working. Having come from New York, I knew little about Boston medicine. I was overjoyed when I learned I'd be starting there. What could be better, I figured, than to begin the year working in a maternity hospital, a place undoubtedly filled with healthy mothers having healthy babies?

It took thirty seconds in the nursery at St. A's to show how wrong I was. Instead of a quiet community hospital where healthy women came to deliver healthy babies, the place was a perinatal referral center, a huge medical pressure cooker. Women from all over New England whose pregnancies had been plagued by serious complications were transferred to St. A's. Sick or premature babies born at smaller hospitals in Massachusetts, New Hampshire, and even Connecticut were transported in. With more than fifty cribs and eighteen ventilator hookups, the neonatal intensive care unit (NICU for short) was a frightening world of high technology, complicated equipment, and some of the smallest, sickest, scariest premature babies anyone could ever imagine.

Looking around the unit that first day, I couldn't even believe that some of those babies were human. None of the fourteen patients in the first two rows had weighed more than two pounds at birth. They were lying naked on devices called warming tables, bathed in bright, fluorescent lights. In a few cases, the tops of the warming tables were covered with pieces of what looked like Saran Wrap, giving the impression that these infants were leftovers, half-eaten chicken wings awaiting refrigeration. Each of the patients was hooked up to a ventilator, and each ventilator made a kind of "siss-pump, siss-pump" sound every time a breath was triggered by the machine's control panel. The cumulative effect of all this was a constant loud rumble on that side of the NICU.

These patients were each covered with intensive care spaghetti, the coiled tubes and wires that attach patients to the machines necessary to sustain their lives. The babies had tubes stuck in their noses and mouths, and intravenous lines in their belly buttons, arms, and legs. Each one was attached to a cardiac monitor lead, with a heat sensor glued onto its chest. In a few cases, I was sure that the equipment needed for intensive care easily outweighed the patient itself. I couldn't believe I was going to spend the next month working in this place, taking care of these patients.

Things looked bad, but they got a lot worse a few minutes later when we started rounds. Ah, my first morning of rounds as an intern, a moment I'd dreamed of for years! I was now going to be able to make a difference in the lives of patients. There was only one problem: I couldn't understand a single word the people running rounds were saying.

Rounds that morning were run by the senior resident (my boss for that month) and the neonatal fellow, a physician who, having completed his residency in pediatrics, was now receiving further training in the care of sick newborn infants. When we stopped at the first bed, the fellow gave us a brief summary of the patient's history: "This is the seven-hundred-gram product of a twenty-six-and-a-half-week gestation born four days ago by C-section for PROM, fetal distress, and a flat tracing. She's got RDS and is on high pressures, like thirty-five over ten, and she's now on an FIO2 of seventy, with a rate of forty. As you can see, she has a UA line and is getting D10W at eighty per kilo per day. We're planning to switch her to TPN in the next day or two, so whoever picks her up will have to do those orders."

He went on like that for another ten minutes, spewing out

abbreviations, lab values, and seemingly random numbers. When he was done, we moved on to the patient in the next bed, and he began the routine all over again. I understood virtually nothing of what he said. All I knew was that some of these babies were being assigned to me. Somehow after rounds, I was expected to take care of them.

There were three interns starting that day. About half an hour into rounds, I asked one of my co-interns, a guy named Ray who had come to Boston from Chicago, if he had any idea of what was going on. "Are you crazy?" he asked. "I haven't understood a word this guy's said since 'Good morning.'" Ray suggested we leave rounds and go get a drink.

It was about 8:30 in the morning.

Though similar to the start of my internship, the experiences of Scott, Hal, and Denise also differed in some ways. Although Scott Lindsay and Hal Burkins were both, like me, graduates of Albert Schweitzer, they had chosen to stay in the Bronx for their residency training. As a result, neither needed to adjust to a new environment that had made my first months so difficult.

Scott also spent his first rotation in a neonatal intensive care unit. On June 30, 1994, the night before beginning the year, he made an entry in his audio diary. His concerns about starting in the NICU were exactly the same as mine had been fifteen years before:

I'm packing up my stuff, getting ready for my first day in the hospital. I chose pediatrics in the first place because I like interacting with kids, and now I'm wondering what it's going to be like to have the babies in the NICU as patients. They're the farthest things from interactive you can get. If these kids even move, it's a bad sign. Moving means there's something wrong with them, like they're having a seizure or something. They move, and we wind up doing a sepsis workup.

I was nervous tonight, knowing that I'd have to get up at six tomorrow morning and get to the hospital. I really wanted to be in bed by ten, but I figured this was my last night of freedom, so I went over to my girlfriend Renee's apartment and we went out. We got some frozen yogurt and talked a little about the challenges our relationship was likely to face during the next few months. I won't be around a lot, and when I am around, there's a good chance I'm going to be tired and cranky. Renee says she's prepared to deal with it. We'll see.

I'm not looking forward to this; I'm really tense. There's a knot in my stomach. I've got to try to get to sleep.

Unlike Scott and Hal, Denise Powers suffered some of the same dislocation I experienced in Boston. At the start of her internship, Denise left her mother, family, and friends in Brooklyn to move to the Bronx. It may have been only a few miles, but it created a gulf larger than had ever before existed between Denise and her loved ones.

Denise's world went through a major transformation. Moving to the Bronx meant finding an apartment and buying furniture, carpeting, and even a car. Methodically, she went down the list of needs, finding an apartment two miles north of Mt. Scopus, our main teaching hospital. She went from store to store buying what she needed and arranging to have it delivered.

Each of these purchases caused at least a minidrama in Denise's already complicated life, similar to my own crisis with United Van Lines. The car she bought, a used Toyota, was a lemon; in fact, at one point in her diary, Denise said she was thinking of having the thing painted yellow, so it would finally resemble what it actually was. Since she'd bought the car in Brooklyn, she wound up spending most of her free time during July and August traveling back and forth between the dealer's garage and her apartment, driving the suspect car one way and taking public transportation the other.

And when she wasn't arguing with the used car dealer in Brooklyn, she was yelling at the dispatcher at one furniture store or another. None of the furniture deliveries came off as planned. Every item took weeks, multiple phone calls, and hours of wasted time waiting for promised deliveries that never arrived.

Denise Powers was a very different person from me. Growing up in the inner city, living with the kind of discrimination she received from the merchants with whom she dealt, she seemed unfazed by the start of internship. On July 1, she walked into Jonas Bronck Hospital, strode onto the general pediatric ward, and picked up her patients. She did her work without any fuss and got out at a reasonable hour. What did she do that evening? Stayed home waiting for the delivery men to bring her new couch. Predictably, they never showed.

Part 2: That First Night on Call

> *Saturday was my first day on call. At around noon, I got paged to pick up an admission in the emergency room. That was the first time I got lost. I couldn't believe it, I wound up wandering around the basement of the hospital for twenty minutes, having no idea where I was. I found the morgue, I found the engineering department, but the ER seemed to be missing. . . . I finally found a guy down there who spoke at least a little bit of English, and I*

asked him where the ER was. He laughed at me for a few minutes and then told me I was on the wrong floor; the ER was one flight up. . . .

I got six admissions during the day and two more in the middle of the night. There were IVs falling out all over the ward that needed to be restarted and hours and hours worth of scut that needed to be done. I got no sleep, I didn't even have a chance to think about lying down, but somehow I made it through and nobody died. So I guess, all in all, I'd have to say it was a successful night. My only problem is, I don't ever want to be on call again.

Mark Greenberg, July 1, 1985

Most interns remember their first night on call for the rest of their lives. Having to stay up all night is not all that unique or unusual. At some point, most people will do it at least once. What's different about being on call as an intern is that not only are you awake and functioning hour after hour, but you're responsible for a fairly large number of human lives. The actions you take, the decisions you make, the details you remember and those you forget have the potential to alter the course of the lives of your patients. And although there's a resident on call with you, the intern is the one writing the nurses' orders: You're the one interpreting the results of blood tests; you're the one starting the IVs and doing the procedures. For all intents and purposes, the buck stops with you.

Like Mark Greenberg, most people survive their first night on call relatively unscathed. For most new doctors, much of that first night—in fact, most of internship—is spent (wasted, in most interns' opinion) in performing the mundane, repetitive tasks called "scut work." But even during their premiere night on call, interns can be thrust into horrible emergency situations. Without doubt, the worst first-night-on-call experience belongs to Andrea Goodman, a woman who did her internship at Jonas Bronck Hospital in 1982. Andrea's story has become legendary in the Bronx. Although it sounds more like fiction than fact, it really happened. I've not only heard the story from Andrea herself, but from two other people who played roles in the experience.

Like Scott Lindsay and me, Andrea Goodman had the bad fortune to begin her internship in the NICU. At 2:20 on the morning of her first night on call, Andrea and her resident, Julie Nathan, were called stat to the Jonas Bronck delivery suite. When they arrived, they were told that a woman who'd received no prenatal care had wandered in off the street in active labor. The obstetric intern explained that although according to the reported first day of her last menstrual period she was only at thirty weeks of gestation (in which case the baby would be ten weeks premature), on examination, her fundal height (the size of her uterus) was forty centimeters, suggesting she was at full term. "Either her dates are off," the obstetric intern told Andrea and Julie, "or she's carrying premie twins or triplets. Since she's never had an ultrasound, we can't tell."

This was not good news: Premie twins or triplets require a great deal of expert care and attention. Although Julie was technically a senior resident, she had only the week before finished her junior residency year. As such, she had only limited experience managing premies and had never been called on to care for two or three sick babies simultaneously. On top of this, Andrea, having never been on call before and being a complete stranger to the neonatal side of the delivery room, would be of little, if any, help.

So, nervously, at 2:25 A.M., the two pediatric residents took their places alongside the infant warming table, the device onto which the baby (or babies) would be plopped following delivery. Julie went through the mental checklist that had to be completed before the birth of any potentially critically ill newborn: She turned up the heat to assure that the surface of the table would be warm enough to prevent the newborn from becoming hypothermic; by twisting a valve, she turned on the room's oxygen supply and attached fresh, sterile tubing to the nipple that protruded from the wall; she removed an ambu-bag (a balloon-like device used to force oxygen into the lungs of sick newborns), a suction catheter, an umbilical artery catheter (a very thin piece of plastic tubing that would be inserted into the artery in the umbilical cord), and some syringes from their sterile packages, placing them on the warming table; and then she drew up the medications that would be used in case the baby or babies required immediate emergency resuscitation. By 2:30, having completed these tasks, Julie and Andrea began to wait for the delivery.

As it turned out, they'd be waiting for a while. The woman, who spoke only Spanish and looked like a teenager, had been placed on the table in the delivery room. Like clockwork, her contractions came every two minutes, and as each contraction reached its peak, she screamed and cursed in Spanish at the top of her lungs. Then, as the pain subsided, she drifted off to sleep for a few seconds, only to have her rest interrupted by the arrival of the next wave of pain.

But the baby refused to come out. From across the room, Andrea could see the top of its head peek through the birth canal. With every contraction, the obstetric intern would yell, "*Puha, señora, puha,*" and the woman would try her best to push the baby out. Again and again, nothing happened.

"The baby's head was clearly out," Andrea told me later. "We could see the hair, we could see the face. Julie even suctioned the nose out with a bulb syringe. But then nothing else happened. We stood there, ready and waiting, but the baby was just stuck."

He *was* stuck. The obstetric intern did everything he knew how to do, but being his first night on call, his repertoire was pretty limited. He pulled on the baby's head; it wouldn't budge. He pushed on the baby's head, trying to get it back up into the uterus; again, nothing happened. At 2:45, after a little more than twenty minutes of trying, now sweating profusely and white as a sheet, the intern called for backup.

The obstetric resident who was covering swaggered in and, with the confidence gained by a whole year of delivering hundreds of babies, set to work. Skillfully, he twisted the head to the left; the baby's position did not change. Next, he twisted the head to the right; again, no movement occurred.

Now, with more force than the intern had used, the resident pulled sharply on the baby's head; it budged not an inch. The resident tried to push the head back up into the birth canal and again nothing happened. He even had the intern sit on the woman's belly and push with all his might at the back of the uterus while he twisted and turned and tried to pull the baby out. There was still no response. "I don't understand what's happening," the resident, sounding less confident now, said to the intern. "This baby seems to be wedged in."

At a little after 3:00, having worked for twenty minutes and done everything he'd been trained to do, the obstetric resident finally admitted defeat. Reluctantly, he asked the nurse to page the perinatal fellow, the most senior obstetrician in the hospital at that hour.

Andrea told me later that while this was happening, she was feeling completely helpless. "Here I am, it's my first night on call, I don't know anything about neonatology, I know very little about obstetrics, but I knew something was terribly wrong. We knew there might be problems from the beginning, but as all that time was passing, every time that woman started screaming at the start of another contraction, we realized whatever was wrong was probably getting worse. And neither of us could do anything to help."

Having been asleep in the on-call room in another part of the hospital, it took the perinatal fellow at least ten minutes to get to the delivery suite. By 3:15, the time he finally reached the delivery room, more than forty-five minutes had passed since the neonatal team had begun waiting. It had been more than half an hour since the baby's head had been delivered.

The perinatal fellow set to work. With a fierceness that came from the understanding that he was the end of the chain, that there was no one more senior to call, he did everything he could to extract that baby: With all his might, he pushed and pulled. At no point was there any movement. With the resident sitting on the woman's abdomen and pushing as forcefully as he could, the perinatal fellow pulled and twisted and yanked and flexed, yet nothing happened. "Call anesthesia," he yelled, recognizing there was something terribly wrong with the situation.

The anesthesiology resident arrived and, without hesitation, put the woman out. When he was sure she was unconscious, the perinatal fellow twisted the head so violently that it appeared as if he might rip it from the baby's neck. It still didn't budge.

And then, he tried again. This time, it worked.

"That's the last thing I remember," Andrea told me. "One second, he was jerking the head, and the next second, the whole thing came off in his hands. I saw him there, holding the separated head, and I just passed out. I'd never fainted before, but there was nothing I could do. My legs just gave out on me."

Realizing that the fetus had become irreparably stuck,

wedged into its mother's pelvis with its head delivered through the birth canal and its body unable to pass through the cervix, and that after more than half an hour without any oxygen going to its brain, the baby was already dead, the perinatal fellow made the only choice that made sense. He decapitated the baby and pushed the now free body back up into the uterus. After placing the lifeless head into a sterile basin, he and the resident performed a cesarean section. After they opened the woman's abdominal wall and entered her uterus, the problem that had led to this disastrous outcome became immediately clear.

What happened in the delivery room that night in July 1982 could never happen at Jonas Bronck Medical Center today. With the placement of ultrasound machines in delivery suites in most major hospitals around the United States, a woman such as this one, arriving in labor with no prenatal care, would receive an immediate sonogram. If that had been done for this patient, it would have been immediately obvious that this fetus could not possibly have been delivered through the birth canal. Affected with a condition known as polycystic kidney disease, a rare, lethal genetic disorder in which the kidneys become immensely enlarged, this fetus's abdominal circumference measured over forty-five centimeters, about ten centimeters larger than the fetal head.

To me, the most amazing fact about Andrea Goodman's first night on call was that it was not her last. Following her syncopal episode, Andrea was tended to by Julie Nathan who, much happier caring for a twenty-five-year-old adult than a set of thirty-week premature triplets, had her intern back on her feet in a matter of minutes. Once out of the delivery room, Andrea went on with her night on call as if nothing had happened. "I don't know exactly how we do it," she said, echoing a thought I've heard again and again. "Once stuff like that happens, you kind of put it out of your head and go on to the next item on your scut list. I guess we're just too busy to think about things for very long."

Regardless of the misery they might encounter during that first night on call, most interns react the way Andrea Goodman did. Somehow, they're able to put the events of the night before out of their minds and return to work the next morning, quickly settling in to the day-to-day grind that becomes their lives. In fact, I know of only one person who, following his first night on call, decided he'd had more than enough internship to last him a lifetime.

One of the smartest people I've ever met, Art Evans came to the Schweitzer School of Medicine from MIT, where he'd amassed a nearly perfect grade point average and Medical College Admission Test scores. Amazingly, Art, who was a classmate of mine, lived in Boston during the first two years of medical school, managing to take the first two years of our medical school curriculum as a kind of correspondence course.

How he did it was staggering. Art would come to New York at the start of each new course, pick up a copy of the syllabus (the annotated lecture notes on which the final exam would be based), then head back to Boston, where he had a full-time job as a computer programmer. Spending most of his free time in a small apartment in Cambridge, Art would return to the Bronx on the day before the scheduled exam. At Schweitzer, he shared an apartment with Jim Richards, one of our classmates. He and Jim would have a leisurely dinner, Jim would fill Art in on some of the gossip, then Art would go into his room and read the syllabus. He'd read it only once, then head off to bed. The next morning, he'd show up to take the exam. Using this approach, Art not only passed every course, he actually managed to get honors in a few of them.

By necessity, Art's life changed drastically when our third year of medical school began. As third-year students, we essentially lived on the wards of the hospital, rotating through each of the major medical specialties. Since passing depended not on exam grades but on our actual performance working with house officers and patients, Art found that to survive, he had to quit his job in Boston, give up his apartment in Cambridge, and move to the Bronx. It was a sacrifice, but Art felt it was probably worth it.

The only problem was that during his rotations, Art found that he enjoyed virtually nothing about clinical medicine. During surgery, he found he hated the macho attitudes of the surgeons; in pediatrics, he discovered he absolutely detested children; while in internal medicine, working with old people bothered him. He found radiology boring and psychiatry frightening. In fact, the only specialty he found he could tolerate was obstetrics and gynecology, and the only reason he enjoyed this field was that he got along well with the doctor who served as his course leader.

So at the start of our fourth year of medical school, when it was time to decide to which residency programs he'd apply, Art, by default, chose OBS/GYN. And on Match Day in March of that year, he found out he'd be spending the next four years working at the OBS/GYN residency program at the University of Pittsburgh.

After graduation in early June, Art left the Bronx reluctantly. It wasn't that he'd come to love the Bronx so much; rather, it was because the thought of living in Pittsburgh made him ill. But Art managed to make the move, and on July 1, he began his training at Pittsburgh's University Hospital.

Art started on the GYN service. His first day went fairly well: He went on rounds with a senior resident, assisted an attending physician with a hysterectomy, spent the afternoon in clinic, and wound up getting out of the hospital before 6:00 P.M. Not exactly thrilled with the work, he found it no more taxing than his rotation during the third year of medical school. The first day went fine; it was the second day that caused Art most of his trouble.

Art was scheduled to be on call the second night of the year. Before the night began, he wasn't too worried. He knew that by having GYN as his first rotation, he'd lucked out. A service with few emergencies and a patient population made up largely of women admitted for hysterectomies and other elective operations, Art knew that GYN was usually quiet at night. At most hospitals, night call for the resident covering the service was composed of working up a few women who were being admitted for surgery the next morning and delivering post-op care to women who had had surgery earlier that day. So Art was prepared for a quiet, laid-back first night experience; he expected to get a fair amount of sleep.

But like my expectations about starting internship at St. Ann's, Art's idea of what a night on call might be like was absolutely wrong. There was one aspect of his job of which he had not been made aware, one role the GYN resident on night call played that would alter the course of Art Evans's life.

At that time, the GYN service at the University of Pittsburgh was a leading center for second-trimester abortions. Women from all over the area who had decided to terminate their pregnancies after the twelfth week were referred to University Hospital for management. Laminaria, a sponge-like substance that causes the cervix to dilate, was implanted into these women's vaginal vaults, and Prostaglandin, a drug that induces contractions, was administered. The women were then placed in private rooms where they would go into labor and eventually deliver dead fetuses.

It turned out that the GYN intern on call was responsible for the management of these women. It was, therefore, Art's job to take care of any complications that might occur. And complications were one thing of which these patients had plenty.

That first night, Art found himself responsible for five patients in various stages of aborting. Three of them were reacting badly to the Prostaglandin. They became so ill, were vomiting so violently, that Art feared they might tear their esophagi. Not knowing exactly what to do, he called the junior resident who was covering him. "Sorry to bother you," he said when he got the resident on the phone, "but all these abortion patients are vomiting their brains out."

"Yeah," the resident said. "So why are you calling me?"

"What am I supposed to do for them?" Art asked.

"Get them to stop," the resident said. "You need me to tell you that?"

"No, I know I'm supposed to get them to stop," Art responded. "I'm calling to find out the best way to do that."

"What are you, a moron?" the resident asked. "You don't know how to get a patient to stop vomiting? My mother knows how to get patients to stop vomiting, and she never went to medical school. You did go to medical school, didn't you?"

Not answering the question directly, Art instead asked, "Is any one antiemetic better than any other?"

"Give them each a shot of Compazine, for God's sake. And don't bother me again with such stupidity." The resident then hung up.

Muttering to himself, Art ordered Compazine for the vomiting patients and tried to finish the rest of his work. But as he was writing progress notes on the three vomiting patients, one of the nurses came up to him and said, "Ms. Smith expelled her fetus ten minutes ago."

"Great news," Art replied.

"The placenta hasn't delivered," the nurse went on. "It hasn't separated."

"So?" Art asked, already figuring something nasty was going to happen.

"I think it needs to be manually extracted."

In those days, this was not an unusual complication of Prostaglandin abortions. Because of the technique, the afterbirth would remain attached to the wall of the uterus following delivery of the fetus. The only way to safely complete the abortion was for the doctor to reach into the uterus and gently tear the placenta away from the uterine wall. It was not a nice job, but it had to be done. And Art was the one who had to do it.

Having never manually extracted a placenta, Art figured he'd check with his resident again. He approached the phone a little more reluctantly this time. "I've got an unseparated placenta," Art said when the resident, who was already in bed in his on-call room, picked up the phone.

"Yeah," the resident said. "So?"

"What do I do?" Art asked.

"Extract it," the resident said.

"How do I do that?" Art asked.

"How do you think you do that?" the resident asked back.

"I would think I should reach into the uterus and separate it from the uterine wall," Art said.

"And they told me you were untrainable!" the resident replied. "I knew there'd be hope for you, Dr. Evans."

"Is there anything special I need to know before I stick my hand up there?" Art asked.

"I'd advise you to wear a glove," the resident replied. "And it's probably not a bad idea to wash your hands after you're done." He then slammed down the phone.

Now cursing to himself, Art followed the nurse into Ms. Smith's room. The room was dark, and the nurse turned on the lights. Having already been placed in the lithotomy position with her feet up in the stirrups, Ms. Smith was crying softly. As the nurse took her place alongside the woman, Art said hello, then went directly to the foot of the bed. He found a metal basin in which a five-inch-long fetus lay. Sitting on the stool, he glanced up at the woman's vagina, from which a thin, torn umbilical cord protruded.

After pulling on a glove, Art probed into the birth canal. The cervix was still dilated enough to allow his hand to pass through. As his hand followed the umbilical cord, which served as a kind of guide wire, up into the uterus, Ms. Smith's crying increased. "This might hurt a little," Art said, almost as an afterthought.

Art's hand found the placenta. Trying to work his fingers into the seam between the afterbirth's membranous covering and the uterus's muscular wall, he found that they seemed to be cemented together. "Uh-oh," he said softly.

"What's wrong?" the nurse asked.

"I can't get it to separate cleanly."

"Well, whatever you do, don't tear it," the nurse ordered. "If you tear it, she'll bleed out."

Art knew this to be the case. Not only did he have to peel the placenta from the wall of the uterus without tearing it, he had to remove every last part of it. His fingers probed the afterbirth from all angles; none of it would give cleanly. After moving his hand around the woman's uterus for nearly ten minutes, he extracted his hand. Excusing himself, he went back to the nurses' station and picked up the phone.

The resident picked up on the fifth ring. "What now?" he asked.

"I can't get the placenta to separate cleanly," he said.

"Now there's a surprise," the resident responded.

"What do you mean?" Art asked.

"If the placenta were ready to separate cleanly, it would have come out with the fetus. It's not mature enough to be separated. You've got to rip it off."

"Rip it off? Won't the patient bleed out?"

"No," the resident responded, "not likely. She might, but it's not likely. Look, just do it and get it over with. And try not to bother me again, okay?" And once again, he hung up.

Within a couple of minutes, terrified now that this woman was going to exsanguinate before his eyes, Art had his hand back in Ms. Smith's uterus. As the woman continued to sob, the intern gingerly tugged on the placenta. Unevenly, his hand felt it give up its hold on the uterine wall. Suddenly, he felt his glove become all wet; pulling his hand out, he found that the glove was covered with bright red blood. Ashen, he stuck his hand back up and, without hesitation, pulled on the placenta with greater force. In a short time, it was free. After throwing it into the metal basin next to the fetus, he reached back into the uterus to check for gushing blood. Although there seemed to be red liquid everywhere, he couldn't find any obvious actively bleeding sites. Using gauze, he mopped up the uterus as best he could. The blood did not reaccumulate.

He had done it: The placenta was out and Ms. Smith had apparently survived. With a deep breath, Art turned his attention to the placenta. Rolling it around in his hands, he saw that it appeared to be present in its entirety. Apparently, nothing had been retained in the uterus.

Ripping off his gloves and disposing of them in the trash,

Art said good night to Ms. Smith. After washing up, he was returning to the nurses' station to write a note in Ms. Smith's chart when a second nurse approached him. "Ms. Jones just delivered her fetus," she said.

With a sharp, stabbing pain suddenly developing in the middle of his gut, Art asked, "And the placenta?"

"It hasn't separated."

Groaning, Art followed the nurse into this patient's room. Ms. Jones had been one of the patients who'd been vomiting heavily from the Prostaglandin, and her room had that sour smell of vomitus. After saying hello, Art replayed the scenario that had occurred minutes earlier with Ms. Smith.

Once again, after he'd succeeded, Art returned to the nurses' station. And once again, almost immediately, he was greeted by another nurse with news that a third patient had failed to expel a placenta.

By this time, Art had had it. Throwing his hands in the air, he said, "That's it." Picking up the phone, he once again called the resident who, by this time, was sound asleep. "What now?" the resident asked, drowsily. "Have you forgotten the dose of aspirin?"

"No, genius, I remember the dose of aspirin," Art began. "I remember just about everything I need to know, including what it means to act like a human being, which appears to be something you either forgot or never learned in the first place. You are a fucking jackass, and as far as I'm concerned, you can fuck yourself and go to hell!"

The resident, realizing that his intern had flipped out, said, "Art, are you okay?"

"Yeah, I'm fine. But there's a woman up here who needs to have a placenta extracted, and I'm not doing it. I'm not doing anything except packing up my junk and getting my ass out of this shithole. I quit! From now on, you're the intern, you piece of excrement!"

And with those words, Art slammed down the phone and ended his career as a doctor. Good to his word, he packed up his belongings, left the ward, got into his car, and drove back to Boston, where he resumed his job as a computer programmer. Not only has he never again practiced medicine, after his few hours on call, he has never regretted his decision.

My first night on call in the NICU at St. Ann's was not exactly filled with uplifting experiences, but it in no way compared with the experiences of Andrea Goodman and Art Evans. I'd lucked out; my first night fell on a Friday. Since I worked every third night, this meant I'd have the first weekend off. The plan was that I'd get out of the hospital early on Saturday morning, drive to Logan Airport to pick up Beth, and we'd go home to our apartment and have a great weekend. At least, that's how we'd laid it out on the phone the night before.

I didn't get any sleep on that Friday night. Doug Berkowitz, the senior resident, and I spent every waking minute caring for a sick infant who was born that evening at about 10:00 P.M. The baby had aspirated meconium (the baby's first bowel movement; its presence in amniotic fluid is a sign of potential fetal distress; when present in amniotic fluid, it can be inhaled during the baby's first breath, causing a serious pneumonia) while passing through the birth canal, and had basically been born dead.

Doug and I (but mostly Doug) had done an entire resuscitation in the delivery room. Through Doug's perseverance, we'd managed to bring this dead baby back to life. But the infant was critically ill, and it took all our efforts to get him stabilized in the NICU.

Exhausted, uneasy with how the night had gone, and unhappy with the prospect of ever returning to the NICU, I signed out quickly on Saturday morning and left the hospital for the airport.

I stopped the car at the curb outside the Eastern terminal. I got there a few minutes before Beth's flight was scheduled to arrive, so I sat there, enjoying the peace of the early morning.

After about fifteen minutes, a rush of activity began around me. People, most of them carrying small suitcases, began walking through the electric doors of the terminal and out into the July morning. I searched the entrance for signs of a familiar face. And then, all at once, there she was; I don't think I'd ever been so happy to see anyone.

I got out of the car and fell into her arms just outside the car's passenger door. We embraced long and hard, in total silence, and when the embrace ended, I opened the door for her and got myself back into the car.

"How are you?" she asked. "I missed you so much."

That's when my wall collapsed. I couldn't help it. I was so tired, so drained, that, like a dam breaking, I burst into tears. I sat with my face buried in the steering wheel of the car, crying. I didn't want to be an intern if being an intern meant I'd have to work like this for a whole year. I never wanted to return to St. Ann's. I just wanted to go home to New York and be a medical student forever.

So began Beth's first weekend in Boston. I'm sure she had no clue as to what had happened; she couldn't have understood what I was going through or what I was thinking, but it didn't seem to matter. She put her arms around me and hugged me, telling me everything would be okay. After a while, she moved me to the passenger's seat and drove the car out of the airport toward Watertown. In the parking lot outside our mostly empty apartment, Beth helped me out of the car, took me upstairs, and got me into my sleeping bag. On the floor, I fell asleep almost immediately and slept soundly until 6:00 that evening.

After waking up, I felt a little better. My emotions were back under control. We went out for dinner that night, then came home to our sleeping bags. By Sunday morning, I was nearly recovered, and by Monday, after I dropped Beth off at the Eastern terminal for her return trip to New York, I was again ready to face the premies.

Although I was better, that first night on call in the NICU at St. Ann's had changed me forever. I became a different person, more cynical, less trusting. I'm still trying to return to my preinternship state; after fifteen years, I still haven't made it.

Almost fifteen years to the day after I'd sat at Logan Airport crying in the front seat of my car, Scott Lindsay was finishing his first night on call in the NICU at West Bronx Hospital. At 11:00 P.M. on July 2, 1994, he made the following entry in his diary:

The NICU: What can I say? It's just overwhelming. These kids are so small and so sick that you're walking on eggs all night long waiting for something to happen. Every one of them has the potential to go into full arrest and die at any minute.

There are these horrible, piercing alarms everywhere, attached to everything. There are alarms that go off if the heart rate or respi-

ratory rate drops or rises, or if the oxygen level goes below a certain point. There are alarms that go off if the ventilator isn't working, if the IV pump gets clogged, or sometimes for no reason at all. Every minute another alarm sounds, and you don't know what it is, whether it's a machine or a baby that's malfunctioning. In the NICU, it's hard to tell where the technology ends and the patient begins.

And let me tell you, those alarms stay with you for a long time. I've been out of the hospital for over twelve hours now. I was just washing my face, getting ready to go to bed, and I swore I heard a respirator alarm going off. I turned away from the sink to see where it was coming from, and there was dead silence. So I guess these alarms have already made an impression on my mind.

I got no sleep at all last night. The resident and I spent the entire night treading water: We never managed to finish everything that needed to get done, but we were never too far behind. There's so much scut to do in the NICU: progress notes, starting IVs in veins that are as wide as dental floss, writing complicated orders for TPN [total parenteral nutrition—intravenous feedings for patients who can't take food by mouth]. You never get a chance to stop and think about what you're doing.

And in the middle of all this, we had to drop everything and rush up to the delivery room three times for emergency deliveries. The first two babies did fine. The first had late decels [a heart rhythm suggestive of fetal distress], but all we had to do was dry the baby off, warm her up, and give her a little oxygen, and she was fine. The second one had meconium staining. By the time we got up to the DR, the baby was already out and doing fine. All we had to do was towel off all the shit that was covering him and send him down to the well baby nursery.

The third baby was the worst. It was a twenty-one-weeker, a miscarriage really, with absolutely no chance for survival. The woman had come in off the street in labor. The midwife had tried to stop the labor with medication, but it hadn't worked, and the baby was coming out. They wanted a pediatrician in the delivery room just in case the mother's dates were off and the baby was viable. So the resident told me to go up and take care of it.

The baby was out by the time I got there. It was in an incubator, wrapped up in a towel, so you could just see the face. It looked like a doll. It had no hair, its eyelids were fused, and, because the skin was so thin, you could see all its veins just under the surface. I listened to the chest with my stethoscope: The heart was pumping away, but there were no breath sounds and it wasn't moving at all. It wasn't really alive, but it wasn't dead yet either. So I had to stay there and wait.

The mother was crying. The chart said she had four other kids, and she was twenty-two years old. I didn't say anything to her. Since there was nothing I could do or say that would make any difference, I figured I'd let the obstetric service handle her.

I stayed with the baby for about a half hour. Eventually, the heart rate sort of faded away and then it was over. I declared the baby dead and got up to go.

I felt bad for the mom, but it was hard to feel any actual loss for the patient, because it just didn't seem like a real human. It had never really been alive, so it was kind of hard to grieve its loss. It wasn't as if it had died; it just happened to come out of the oven a little too early.

After coming back from the DR, the night went along without incident. I didn't get any sleep and I was exhausted and felt really crabby, but this morning, I managed to finish my notes, sign out, and leave the hospital by 10:00.

Part 3: The First Month—Making Friends with Patients

For those of us who made it through a first night and were insane enough to return to the hospital the next day for more, life as an intern ultimately settled into a regular routine. The first months of internship turn into something of a dance, a constant negotiation between the newly graduated doctor and the people with whom he or she works: the residents and chief residents who provide support and backup; the nurses and ancillary staff who work as a team to provide care to the patient; and, most important, the patients and their families. When it comes to these relationships, new interns are usually at their best. Still well rested, humble, and thankful for any help, interns are at the top of their psychosocial game. Things are often going so well that it may take them until September or October to get into their first argument with a lab technician.

It's the relationship with patients that is most important in the first few weeks of internship. When it came to dealing with my patients and their families during my first month of internship, I was at something of a disadvantage. One problem with working in NICU is that you can't communicate with your patients. Tiny and sick, they can't tell you what hurts, when it hurts, or why it hurts. And because St. Ann's was a referral center accepting transfers from all over New England, many of the parents and families of my patients simply could not visit more than once a week.

Of the three interns who started in July 1994, Hal Burkins had the best opportunity to bond with his patients. He began his internship on the adolescent unit at Mt. Scopus Medical Center, a ward filled with teenagers having an assortment of chronic and acute diseases. During his first month, Hal befriended Angela Park, a fourteen-year-old girl, and her family. Angela, who was transferred to Hal's service on the first day of the month, had only days before been diagnosed with an unusual type of non-Hodgkins lymphoma, a cancer of the lymphatic system. Angela came to adolescents' from the intensive care unit, where she'd initially been admitted to begin her first course of chemotherapy. Here are entries from Hal's diary:

July 4, 1994 [after his first night on call]

Angela Park, my fourteen-year-old patient with lymphoma, is the daughter of a physician. She's a sweet, intelligent kid, and unfortunately she knows exactly what's going on with her medical condition. I feel really bad for her; I can't imagine what it's like being fourteen and knowing you have cancer.

Angela had a rocky course in the beginning, but she seems to be stable now. Although she's still very sick, she's really a terrific kid. When I examined her belly this morning, she couldn't stop giggling, because she's so ticklish. I kept doing it, and she kept laughing. That was the first time I was able to get any kind of a smile out of her. I just can't understand how this can happen to someone.

July 8

Angela continues to improve. She had a repeat CT scan yesterday; it showed that the tumor had shrunk so much that it was almost gone. That was great news.

Although Angela's better, dealing with her father has become more difficult. The father is a doctor on staff at Mt. Scopus, and he's incredibly overbearing. He has his nose in the girl's chart practically every day. Dr. Edelstein, our attending this month, pointed out on rounds that since he works here, he has access to all the girl's lab values via the hospital's computer system, too. This is a real problem: There are things the family needs to know and there are things that should be private and privileged information between Angela and her doctors. Dr. Edelstein gave me specific instructions that the father is not allowed to look at Angela's chart, that it is not a public document open for everyone to read. I agree with him completely.

The discussion we had on rounds about access to the chart encouraged me to go and have a talk with Angela. As usual, her mother was with her when I got there. Her mother's always with her. She spends day and night with the girl. But unlike the father, the mother is very considerate of Angela's privacy. Every time I come into the room to examine Angela or talk with her, the mother makes a point of getting up and leaving.

Anyway, after Mrs. Park left the room, I took a seat at Angela's bedside. She's very shy, very reserved, and she's not willing to express her feelings or emotions to someone like me, who's considered an outsider. I asked her if she knew that her father had access to all the records. She said she did know. I explained that she should not be intimidated by that, that if there were private things she wanted to say or needed to tell me, I would keep them secret and not put them in the chart. She didn't say anything, she just nodded her head. But I know she understood what I was talking about. Hopefully, she'll eventually feel comfortable enough to confide in me.

Mrs. Park has let me know, in a few subtle ways, that she likes and trusts me. Knowing this has made me want to do a better job in taking care of her daughter. It's funny. As an intern, when you first get a new admission, the patient is nothing more than an anonymous pile of work. You have to write a note, start an IV, draw blood, write orders, check the lab results, and do a lot of other things. To the family, of course, this anonymous pile of work is a very important person, a beloved daughter or son whose illness affects every aspect of that family's life. It takes a while before those feelings get through to the intern. It's starting to happen to me with Angela now.

July 20

Angela has clearly become my favorite patient. She's much better than she was at the start of the month. As a result of the chemotherapy she's received, she became very anemic, and it seemed as if all the life had gone out of her. We wanted to give her a transfusion days ago, but her father wouldn't give his consent. He was afraid she'd get hepatitis or AIDS. But he finally consented, and we gave her two units of packed red cells yesterday and now she's back to her old self again. It was nice to see her walking around the ward. It was as if her life had come back into her. It's amazing what a little blood can do for you. I think it's even made her less depressed.

Unfortunately, we got some of the lab tests back and it turns out that her cancer is more aggressive than was originally thought. Because of this, her chemotherapy was changed to a more intensified protocol. So even though she's feeling better and her tumor has shrunk down to nearly nothing, she's in for a rough road ahead.

The Parks have become much more kind and warm with me. The mother always insists that I be the one to draw Angela's blood when she needs blood tests done. She trusts me, and that's done a lot for my self-confidence.

July 24

Good news: Angela Park's cancer is officially in remission. She had a bone marrow biopsy, and it showed that her marrow has responded beautifully to the chemotherapy and is now producing normal white blood cells. Angela's feeling much better, her spirits are up, and she's scheduled to go home on leave from the hospital this weekend. That's really great news.

I've gotten to be good friends with her mother. The other day, the mom brought me a tape of Angela playing the cello. It was amazing. It turns out that Angela is an exceptionally talented cellist. She's a member of the Westchester Youth Orchestra, and she was selected to audition for the National Youth Orchestra, which is very prestigious. She's scheduled to audition in November, but it's unclear at this point whether she'll be well enough to go.

I tried to convince Angela to have her mother bring her cello to the hospital so she could play while she's an inpatient. She was completely against that. Later on, when I asked her mother about it, she told me that Angela's a real perfectionist and that since she hasn't played in over a month and because her fingers are still tingling, which is a side effect of her chemotherapy, she just wouldn't feel comfortable doing it.

Dr. Goodwin, the oncologist, came to talk to Angela's parents today. He and Dr. Park have an interesting relationship. It turns out that not only is Angela's father a physician, he's actually an oncologist. So Dr. Goodwin can "talk the talk" with him. In order to get a second opinion, Dr. Park actually went to Memorial/Sloan-Kettering and presented Angela's case at the tumor board. He came back satisfied, because they basically came to the same conclusion that Dr. Goodwin had, that Angela needed more intensified chemotherapy. So they're going to give her this week-

end off, and then she'll come back into the hospital on Monday and start on more powerful drugs. The poor kid is going to wind up getting really sick.

I noticed today that Angela's hair is beginning to fall out. She's clearly aware of it, there was hair all over her pillow when I went in to draw her blood this morning. She didn't say anything about it, but she clearly knows what's going on.

I've had to draw blood from all the members of the family for HLA studies. If any of them match Angela's HLA types, they may be able to do a bone marrow transplant.

I'm leaving the service in a few days. I don't mind leaving adolescents', but it is going to be hard to leave Angela. She's really my favorite patient.

All three of the interns made it through the first cycle in good shape: still reasonably well rested, basically happy, and satisfied with their lives. In listening to each of their diaries, I had the impression that they weathered the first month in much better shape than I or even than the interns of *The Intern Blues* had. It seemed as if being on every fourth night instead of every third may actually have made a significant difference.

But internship is more than the first month; the year is twelve rotations long.

2

AUGUST

The Second Rotation: Some Trouble with Attendings

At noon on Monday, August 6, 1979, I sneaked away from attending rounds in the NICU at the Boston Medical Center and headed for the building's lobby. I was post-call that morning, and during the previous night, I'd become paranoid, sure someone was spying on me. I was positive that, somehow, "they" knew that I was planning to do something that interns in the second month of their internships are not supposed to do.

Checking in all directions to make sure I wasn't followed, I entered the mostly deserted lobby at the main entrance to the building. Convinced that no one was watching, I ducked into one of the phone booths, closed the door, picked up the phone, and dialed a number I'd grown familiar with during my years as a medical student in the Bronx. After the secretary answered, I told her who I was and asked to speak to Dr. Cozza.

Alan Cozza, the chief of pediatrics at Jonas Bronck, had been my adviser and friend during my fourth year of medical school. Although he'd encouraged me to stay in the Bronx, in the final analysis, he hadn't thought doing my residency at the Boston Medical Center was such a bad idea. At least, he hadn't tried very hard to talk me out of it.

"Bob," Alan said when he picked up the phone. "How are you doing? How are things going?"

I didn't answer his questions directly. Instead, I responded with a single sentence: "Alan, get me the hell out of here!"

It's unusual for a house officer to decide to leave an internship as early as the first week in August, but I had plenty of reasons for wanting to get out of Boston. Some of them were good, logical, and carefully thought-out. Others were pretty lame, easily solved with little effort during the next few months. But on that Monday morning, none of this mattered. I was miserable, I hated my job and hated my life, and I wanted out.

I'll admit some of my reasons were just situational. The Arab oil embargo dragged on, United Van Lines continued to hold our furniture hostage on a moving truck, and I was still spending my noncall nights trying to sleep in my sleeping bag on the floor of our empty bedroom. Although I'd bought an air mattress (and thinking about it now, probably should have sprung for a cot), I knew that, sometime in the near future, the truck would pull up in front of our building, unload our stuff, and I'd finally be able to get a good night's sleep. But on that Monday, I was overtired and unhappy.

The continuing absence of my wife added to this. Beth was spending weekdays in New York, trying to finish the lab work necessary to complete her dissertation. I knew that at some point she'd finish and join me, but I still felt as if something were missing.

There were other factors making my life miserable, things that had become apparent during the past few weeks that I knew wouldn't get better, problems built into the training program. In August, I spent my second straight month working in a neonatal intensive care unit. Starting an internship at a place like St. Ann's was cruel enough, but then to be assigned the very next month to Children's Four, the NICU at the medical center, was abusive.

I'd come to hate working with premies. Being on call in the NICU amounted to spending thirty-six hours on my feet, running from one disaster to the next. I had gotten virtually no sleep during any of my nights on call, and I'd already stood over and watched at least a half dozen sick babies die.

Take what happened on the afternoon before I placed my call to Alan Cozza. I got a call from Charlie Erickson, the senior resident who was on with me, telling me I was getting a transfer from St. Ann's.

"A transfer from St. A's?" I asked, surprised. "Why would St. A's transfer a patient to us?"

"Something about them being filled up," the resident replied. "Look, the reason doesn't matter. The fact is, the baby's being brought over by the NICU fellow. It's a twenty-six-weeker who was born this morning. He's already intubated, he's got an umbilical artery line in, and they say he's stable."

At least I'd learned something during my six weeks of internship; I knew exactly what Charlie was talking about. I'd spent enough time in the NICU to know exactly what the rest of my on-call day and night was going to be like. This baby was critically ill: I was going to be with him constantly, adjusting his ventilator settings, monitoring his blood for oxygen and carbon dioxide content, fiddling with his fluids to keep his electrolytes in balance, and on and on. The net effect: I would be up all night, and the baby might survive. Only one thing was certain: I wasn't looking forward to the next thirty hours.

I realize now I should have been more suspicious. Having worked at St. A's, I knew their NICU was enormous; in the entire month I'd worked there, the unit had never been too full to take one more baby. I should have realized immediately that this baby was a dump, a term I didn't learn until later in my internship.

At a little after 3:00 P.M., the NICU's doors swung open and the transport team arrived, pushing a portable incubator ahead of them. As the nurses quickly got the baby arranged on a warming table, the fellow from St. A's gave me a very brief run-down of what had been going on. "He's a twenty-six-weeker born at about ten this morning. Birth weight was 520 grams . . . "

"Five hundred and twenty grams!" I repeated, incredulous (520 grams is about 1 pound 2 ounces). I knew that a "normal" twenty-six-weeker should weigh about 800 grams (or a whopping 2 pounds). "You sure this baby's really a twenty-six-weeker?"

Somehow managing to keep a straight face, the fellow replied, "Yup, twenty-six weeks according to the mom's last menstrual period. I guess there's some degree of IUGR [intrauterine growth retardation]. Anyway, the baby's stable, and the medical history's on the transfer sheets. Any questions?"

I could see he was in a hurry, and I couldn't think of anything to ask, so I just shook my head. By this point, the nurses had gotten the baby all set up, and the members of the transport team were reassembling out in the hall. I walked out to say good-bye to the fellow. "Call if you have any questions," he said from inside the elevator as the doors were closing.

As I turned to walk back into the NICU, I heard an alarm go

off. "What?" I managed to ask as the nurse assigned to the brand-new baby said, "Heart rate's below fifty. He's going to arrest."

While yelling for the ward clerk to page Charlie Erickson stat, I rushed to the baby's bedside and got my first good look at him. This baby was minuscule, much smaller than any twenty-six-weeker I'd seen at St. A's, and, frankly, he looked dead. His skin, which had been pink when the transport team arrived, was now ashen gray. He wasn't moving a muscle. Sticking my stethoscope over his chest, I yelled to the nurse, "Did his tube slip?" She shook her head. By then, the baby's heart rate was down to about ten beats per minute, and I couldn't hear breath sounds on either side of the chest.

At this point, the rest of the nursing staff converged on the baby. I yelled for a dose of atropine, a drug that would increase the baby's heart rate. As the nurse was handing me the medication, Charlie Erickson ran into the unit. "What's going on?" he yelled.

"This is the transfer from St. Ann's . . ." I began to explain.

"Why didn't you page me when he got here?" the resident interrupted.

"He just did get here," I answered. "They came, they left, and he immediately arrested." While saying this, I plunged the needle from the syringe holding the atropine through the port in the baby's umbilical artery line and slowly pushed down the plunger. The baby's heart rate responded instantly, coming up to forty in the first few seconds.

Getting closer, Charlie asked, "This is a twenty-six-weeker?"

"That's what the fellow said," I replied, watching the monitor closely. At first, the heart rate climbed, but now it seemed stuck at sixty, less than half of what it should be for a baby of this age. His skin still had that sickly gray pallor.

"This is no twenty-six-weeker," the resident said. Using the thumb and pointer of his left hand, he tried and failed to pry open the baby's eyelids. "Shit," he yelled. "The lids are fused. This baby's less than twenty-four weeks. They've dumped a twenty-four-weeker with a heart rate on our doorstep."

"What do you want to do?" I asked. I knew that in 1979, no baby born prior to twenty-six weeks of gestation had ever survived.

"What's our choice?" he responded. "He's here, and now he's our responsibility. If we do nothing, we'll get nailed on rounds tomorrow. He probably blew a pneumothorax [suffered a collapsed lung]. Let's transilluminate him."

Charlie, who was sure that the pressure with which the ventilator was forcing oxygen into this baby's lungs had caused one of his lungs to collapse, turned out to be right. After darkening the NICU, we shone a bright light onto the baby's chest: The right side lit up like a lightbulb, a sign that air had collected in the chest outside the lung. Telling me to watch closely, Charlie pushed a chest tube into the baby's pleural cavity on that side. Instantly, the baby's heart rate came up to 140 and his skin color changed from gray to pink. As the resident sutured the tube into place, I told him he'd saved the baby's life.

"Terrific," he replied with a snicker. "I saved a twenty-four-weeker. That counts for a lot. I hope you were watching what I did: I have a feeling this isn't going to be the last time this happens with this kid, and the next time, you're putting the tube in."

I was hoping Charlie would be wrong, that it wouldn't happen again, but, unfortunately, I got my chance to pass a chest tube about two hours later. I was sitting in the nurse's station when I heard the cardiac monitor's alarm go off. "He's coding," the nurse yelled. Once again, as I rushed to his side, I shouted for the clerk to page Charlie. By the time he came running through the door of the unit, I was already transilluminating the baby's chest. As it had before, the right side was lighting up.

"Okay," Charlie said. "This one's yours."

Mimicking everything he'd done, I solemnly scrubbed the baby's chest with betadyne soap and covered the region with sterile drapes. After opening the package that held the tube, I pulled on a pair of gloves. "You've got to push really hard," the resident said as he watched my actions approvingly.

Holding the tube over the baby's chest, I pushed. Nothing happened.

"Push harder," Charlie yelled.

"I'll break the baby in half," I yelled back.

"No you won't," Charlie replied. "Push harder and it'll go in."

I pushed harder. Again nothing happened.

"Push with all your might," the resident said. "Don't be a wimp. You're not going to hurt the baby any more than he's already hurting."

Leaning on the tube as hard as I could, I pushed again. This time, I felt a pop as the tube passed through the skin and into the pleural cavity. Once again, almost immediately, the baby's heart rate rose and his color improved dramatically.

I have to admit, successfully passing that chest tube was a terrific feeling. It gave me a feeling of invincibility: For a short time, I believed I could do anything. So, at around 11:00 P.M. when that baby arrested for a third time and I found the left side of his chest transilluminated, I didn't even page the resident. I decided to try a solo flight, to put the third chest tube in by myself.

Once again, I got all set up: I scrubbed the tiny chest with the surgical soap, draped it with sterile sheets, opened the tube's package, and donned the gloves. This time, not afraid I'd do any harm, I placed the sharp end of the tube in the interspace between the fourth and fifth ribs and pushed with all my strength. Once again, I felt that wonderful, rewarding pop.

But this time, rather than immediately rising to over 100, the baby's heart rate plunged. Removing the trochar—the sharp, metal inner portion of the tube—I was greeted with the rush of a stream of blood. "Oh shit," I said, and the nurse who was helping me echoed that comment. I once again yelled for Charlie Erickson to be stat paged, but this time, the resident could do nothing to help the situation.

By jabbing that third chest tube directly into that premature baby's heart, I had instantaneously and unequivocally killed him. When he arrived, Charlie Erickson was almost relieved by this news. "Don't worry about it, Bob," he said. "There was nothing we could've done. This kid was never anything more than a spontaneous abortus: twenty-four-weekers don't have even a one percent chance of surviving. At least you got a chance to learn how to put in a chest tube."

For some reason, the resident's words didn't bring me a whole lot of solace. I stayed awake all that night taking care of all the scut work I'd neglected while involved with this baby. When I did have the chance to reflect, I felt terrible about what I'd done and how that poor baby died.

By the next morning when my relief showed up, I'd already decided I'd had enough of life in Boston. I was depressed, over-tired, and, as I've already mentioned, paranoid. I'd been think-ing about calling Alan Cozza to see if I could line up a job as a second-year resident for the following July, but I hadn't yet definitely made the decision. It was attending rounds that Monday morning that finally pushed me over the edge.

Of course, during rounds I got yelled at for the death. The neonatologists at Boston Medical Center kept careful records of the number of deaths that occurred during their months on service, and having a baby die on your time, regardless of whether the death was preventable or not, was considered a black mark on your record. "I heard a baby died last night," Dr. Moore, the neonatologist, said at the start of rounds. "What happened?"

I reviewed the story for him, from beginning to end. He criticized me six separate times. He said I should have called him at home each time the baby arrested. He didn't like the ventilator settings Charlie and I had put him on (the same ventilator settings, by the way, that the baby had been on when the neonatal fellow from St. Ann's dropped him off). He said that I should never have taken it upon myself to pass a chest tube without supervision. I didn't argue with him; I was too tired and angry, and I figured it would only get me into trouble.

The real problem occurred a few minutes later. We'd actually begun rounding on the living patients and were standing at the bedside of an infant who'd been born a few days before, a twenty-nine-weeker who was on a ventilator. Dr. Moore began fiddling with the machine's controls. We remained in silence as he worked, but I was interested in finding out what he was doing, so I finally asked, "Excuse me, Dr. Moore, what are you trying to achieve?"

The attending, still silent, continued to fiddle with the knobs and buttons.

Thinking he hadn't heard me, I asked again. "Excuse me, Dr. Moore, but what are you trying to achieve by adjusting the ventilator?"

Still playing with the machine's controls, he again remained silent. I was starting to think the poor guy might have a hearing problem so, raising my voice, I repeated the question for the third time: "Dr. Moore," I nearly yelled, "what are you trying to achieve with the ventilator?"

This time, the attending looked up from the dials. "Look," he said, fixing his gaze directly on my face, "attending rounds are reserved for caring for the patients. There is no time for teaching during attending rounds. By asking these questions, you're destroying my concentration. Please be quiet and speak only when I ask you a direct question. If we have time after I'm finished, I'll be more than happy to answer your questions."

I was stunned. I'd never seen nor heard of an attending physician telling an intern that teaching wasn't one of the goals of rounds. Teaching house officers about the management of the patients under their care so that they might be able to function as attending physicians in the future was the main reason for having a residency training program. By shunting this responsibility aside, ignoring my question, and actually yelling at me for asking it, Dr. Moore had succinctly summarized the philosophy of residency training that pervaded the Boston Medical Center's pediatric department.

I remained quiet during the rest of the time we spent walking around, at least until I felt comfortable escaping to the phone booth. That morning's attending rounds with Dr. Moore confirmed my decision: I needed to get out of the Boston Medical Center as soon as possible.

After hearing me out that morning, Alan Cozza sympathized with my plight and offered some words of encouragement, but he also told me it was far too soon to know whether there'd be any openings in the Jonas Bronck program the following July. He did make me a promise, however: "Bob, if there's even a chance we'll have an open spot, you've got the job. Just hang in there!"

A few weeks later, while I was still struggling with life in the NICU, Alan called to give me the good news: One of the Jonas Bronck interns was getting married to a man in Boston; she had informed Alan she was going to leave, and Alan offered me her place. In fact, that intern and I wound up trading places the next year. We both agreed that I got the best of that deal.

A house officer having a bad experience with an attending physician is not all that shocking. You'd think that being on the same team, these two groups would have overlapping agendas. There are, however, many competing issues between attending physicians and house officers that are bound to create friction. The main goal of the intern is to get to sleep. In order to reach this goal, the doctor-in-training must get scut work done as quickly as possible, pacify the nursing staff so that they believe everything that needs to be done has been done, and get patients' needs squared away so they won't nag the staff all night.

The attendings, however, have an entirely different set of goals that revolve mainly around public relations issues. In addition to trying to get their patients well, they also need to keep them happy and satisfied. They also want to keep the hospital's administration happy. While in many cases, these desires on the part of the house staff and attending staff dovetail nicely, there are other times when they significantly conflict.

An amazing example of this occurred at Mt. Scopus in the summer of 1984. New York was in the grip of a strike by Local 1199, the union to which most of the hospital workers belonged. As a result of the strike, many normal hospital services were severely curtailed: The custodians were picketing, so there was no one to clean the wards and empty the trash; the attendants were out, so the job of transporting patients to the X-ray department, therapy sessions, and the operating rooms fell on the medical students, interns, and residents; and the lab technicians were out, so the hospital's administration ordered the attending staff to try to keep lab tests to a minimum.

Prior to performing an operation, in order to assure that the patient is not affected with any underlying condition that would endanger his or her chances of survival, hospitals require certain tests. Before going to the OR, it's routine practice to perform a chest X ray, complete blood count (to assure the patient is not anemic and does not have leukemia), bleeding studies (to rule out the presence of a clotting disorder), and a urinalysis or UA (to make sure an infection isn't present). Usually, these tests are done on the night before surgery so that the results are back in the chart before the patient goes to the operating room.

In the summer of 1984, there was a shortage of personnel to perform these routine tests. Neither the chest X ray nor the blood tests were problematic, because they were all automated. But the UAs had to be done by hand, and up in the lab there just weren't enough hands around to do them. In addition, a UA is a test that interns could easily perform: It amounted to dipping a dipstick into the urine, checking for color changes on a chart, and then briefly examining a sample of the urine under a microscope. The whole procedure, from the time the urine specimen is handed to the intern to the time the evaluation is completed, takes no more than ten minutes.

So in early August of that year, Dr. J. Cuthbert Reid, the chairman of surgery, and Dr. Eric Eisen, the director of laboratories at Mt. Scopus, met and agreed that until the end of the strike, the housestaff would be responsible for performing UAs on all pre-op patients. Following the meeting, Dr. Reid sent out a memo to all house officers under his charge detailing the agreement and ordering them to stop sending urine specimens to the lab.

Before proceeding, a few words must be said about J. Cuthbert Reid. A larger-than-life figure who'd been chairman of surgery at Mt. Scopus for more than twenty years, Dr. Reid was an imposing, politically powerful, internationally renowned academician who, among other peculiarities, had an irrational hatred for the members of his own housestaff. Believing house officers were nothing more than indentured servants, he took every opportunity to rub his young colleagues' noses in their lowly status. And J. Cuthbert Reid did not keep these feelings hidden: From his office desk lamp, a GI Joe doll dressed in a surgical scrub suit hung by a well-formed, miniature noose. If you asked Dr. Reid who this doll represented, he answered without hesitation, "My housestaff." To put it simply, this was not a man whose memoranda should be ignored.

As it turned out, though, the housestaff did largely ignore J. Cuthbert Reid's memo about urinalyses. Having been trained to send these specimens to the lab, to do otherwise now proved difficult. In addition, although each test did take only ten minutes, the house officers on the surgery service were already overwhelmed with performing the jobs of union members who were on the picket line. When you have six or seven patients scheduled to go to the OR the next day, those ten minutes can drag into hours of pointless, needless work, proving to be just one more in a long line of obstacles preventing the house officer from reaching his or her ultimate goal, which, once again, is to get to sleep.

So through the first weeks of August, the specimens of urine from pre-op patients kept arriving in the lab for urinalyses, and

Dr. Eisen and his staff continued to have to drop their other tasks and perform these tests themselves. A week after their initial meeting, Dr. Eisen called Dr. Reid to inform him of the situation, and J. Cuthbert Reid promptly ordered the surgery services' four chief residents into his office, where he screamed and yelled at them about "the urinalysis situation," as he called it, for a good ten minutes. At the end of that meeting, J. Cuthbert Reid ordered his chiefs to make sure that from that moment on no additional urine from pre-op patients arrived in the lab.

Unfortunately, the chief residents could not deliver on that order. Like the rest of the housestaff, they believed that forcing the interns to do all those UAs was ludicrous, especially when so many other more serious problems interfered with the delivery of good patient care. As a result, there was no decrease in the flow of urine samples into the lab. A few days later, Dr. Eisen placed another phone call to Dr. Reid, who, by this point, was clearly furious.

The chairman of surgery spent the next few hours plotting his revenge. Sending memos to the housestaff didn't help, he reasoned, because these people apparently were not smart enough to read. And yelling at the chief residents didn't help, because those guys were clearly too intellectually impaired to pass the simple message along to their underlings. No, something dramatic was needed, something that on the one hand would be punitive, but on the other would serve to show how small and worthless the members of the housestaff actually were.

The answer came to J. Cuthbert Reid in an inspired flash. Early the next morning, the department of surgery's weekly grand rounds was scheduled to occur. Dr. Reid figured he'd take advantage of the opportunity to play out his little drama.

•

The next morning, as the faculty and housestaff of the department of surgery entered the auditorium in which grand rounds was held, they found that a table had been set up adjacent to the speaker's podium at the front of the room. On that table, in a neat row, sat four specimen jars filled nearly to the top with a yellow liquid. When everyone had taken a seat, J. Cuthbert Reid called the meeting to order and, after asking the chief residents to come forward, began his diatribe.

"As you all know," he said, addressing the group, "our hospital is in the midst of a strike by Local 1199. As a result of this strike, extraordinary measures have needed to be taken in order to assure the continuation of quality patient care. I'm happy to report that, for the most part, members of our department have done an exceptional job in coping with this unusual turn of events. However, one group has repeatedly let us down. Ten days ago, I sent a memo to all members of the housestaff ordering that until the strike comes to an end, specimens of urine for routine urinalysis not be sent to the hospital's lab. After a week passed, and I was informed by the hospital's director of the laboratories that no appreciable decrease in the number of requests for urinalyses from our department had occurred, I called these four doctors, our chief residents, to my office and ordered them in no uncertain terms to make sure that my original request be carried out. Last night, much to my chagrin, I received yet another call from Dr. Eisen, the director of laboratories, again informing me that the number of requests for urinalyses on preoperative patients had not changed."

Then J. Cuthbert Reid turned his attention to the four chief residents: "Now, as you four are well aware, I'm used to getting what I want, and I'm not happy when people fail me. I've sent memoranda to you, I've spoken to you, I've given you direct orders, and still you did not carry out my command. What am I to do? How can I get across to you that I really mean what I've been saying? Clearly, mere words will not work. So, I've concluded that it's time for action. On the table in front of you, you see four specimens of urine obtained from patients who are scheduled for surgery this afternoon. These specimens were sent by this housestaff to the laboratory last night for routine urinalysis. Having retrieved them from the lab, I have set them out here to teach you a lesson. I now want each of you, in full view of the entire staff, to drink these specimens."

Without moving a muscle below their necks, the chief residents stared at J. Cuthbert Reid as if the man had suddenly gone insane. After a minute, Dr. Reid, growing impatient, began again: "We will not proceed with grand rounds until you accede to my demand. We will stay here all day if you do not obey. You might as well drink these specimens now, so we can get on with our scheduled program."

Three of the chief residents remained in place, their faces red with embarrassment. But one of them—whose face was red with anger, not shame—leapt into action. Still staring at his chairman, Curt Harris approached the table. He picked up one of the specimen cups, raised it to his lips, and drank down the contents (which, incidentally, turned out to be apple juice). Without a word, and to the cheers of the assembled housestaff, Curt then stormed out of the auditorium and headed for the public phone down the hall, where he called one of his friends, a reporter at the *New York Times*. In great detail, Curt told his friend exactly what had just transpired.

The story in the *Times* and the ensuing torrent of bad publicity went a long way to bring the arrogant J. Cuthbert Reid back down to Earth. Although he didn't lose his job, he was forced to apologize to his house officers and to kiss a lot of administrative ass. The whole event served to weaken immensely Dr. Reid's position in the medical community.

I came to know Curt Harris much later, after he'd finished his training in plastic surgery. At the time of the urine-drinking grand rounds, Curt had already been accepted at a plastic surgery residency program and had little to lose by doing what he did. The rest of that academic year was difficult for him, but he survived it. He's older now, but he's told me that if faced with the same situation, he'd do it again in a minute.

The experience I had with Dr. Moore during my August rotation was not all that novel; as long as there have been attendings and house officers, there have been problems between them. Consider this excerpt from Samuel Shem's novel *The House of God*, one of the first books to focus on the insanity of internship. It's the early 1970s, and during his first rotation on the medicine service at the House of God, a Boston teaching hospital, the narrator, an intern named Roy Basch, is on attending rounds (or Visit, as this exercise is referred to at this hospital) with the rest of his team:

> Being an academic house affiliated with the BMS (Best Medical School in the world), the House of God had a Visit for each ward team . . . who held teaching rounds every day. Our Visit was George Donowitz, a Private who'd been pretty good in the prepenicillin era.

The patient presented was a generally healthy young man who'd been admitted for routine tests of his renal function. My BMS, Levy, presented the case, and when Donowitz grilled him about the diagnosis, the BMS, straight from the library of obscure diagnoses, said "amyloidosis."

"Typical," muttered the Fat Man [Basch's resident] as we gathered around the patient's bed, "typical BMS. A BMS hears hoofbeats outside his window, the first thing he thinks of is a zebra. This guy's uremic from his recurrent childhood infections that damaged his kidneys. Besides, there's no treatment for amyloid, anyway."

"Amyloid?" asked Donowitz. "Good thought. Let me show you a bedside test for amyloid. As you know, people with the disease bruise easily, very easily indeed."

Donowitz reached down and twisted the skin on the patient's forearm. Nothing happened. Puzzled, he said something about "sometimes you have to do it a bit harder," and took hold of the skin, wadded it up, and gave a tremendous twist. The patient gave a yelp, leaped off the mattress, and began to cry with pain. Donowitz looked down and found that he'd ripped a big chunk of flesh from the guy's arm. Blood was squirting from the wound. Donowitz turned pale and didn't know what to do. Embarrassed, he took the piece of flesh and tried to put it back, patting it down as if he could make it stay in place. Finally mumbling, "I . . . I'm sorry," he ran out of the room. With a cool expertise, the Fat Man put a gauze compression bandage on the wound. We left.

"So what did you learn?" asked Fats. "You learned

that uremic skin is brittle, and that the House Privates stink. . . . If [the patient] knew about this, it would be Malpractice City."

My situation was unusual. August, September, and October are usually happy times for interns. They've adjusted to their new lives. They're exhilarated and excited by the work, finally feeling they're doing what they've always waited to do, and not yet so worn down that their nerves are frayed. As a result, interns during this time of year usually get along with everybody—attendings, other house officers, nurses, and patients alike.

But the life of an intern is never exactly a party; there are always difficulties. Of the three interns whose progress I followed in 1994, Denise Powers's experience was the closest to my own. New to the program, having problems with the delivery of the new furniture she'd ordered, and having ongoing car trouble, her life seemed destined to fall apart in August. She managed to keep it together, but apparently came pretty close to losing it on more than one occasion.

Unfortunately for her, Denise turned out to be outstanding at finding attending physicians who had trouble understanding her motivation. As a result, there were attendings whom she came to hate with a passion. Some of these attendings wound up hating her in return.

The attending physicians form the faculty of any pediatric department, and at Albert Schweitzer more than four hundred full- or part-time pediatricians have faculty appointments. As would be expected in any large group of people, some of our faculty members are good, caring, concerned physicians who are also great teachers, but some of them are . . . well, let's say they fall a little short of this ideal condition.

To an intern, it only takes bad experiences with one or two attendings to make the internship experience a horror show. Like my difficulty with Dr. Moore, Denise Powers's problems with attendings started in August.

That month, Denise was spending her second rotation at Jonas Bronck Medical Center. During her nights on call, she worked under the leadership of an attending named Erica Cintron. To say that Denise and Erica didn't exactly hit it off would be something of an understatement. Here are some excerpts from Denise's diary:

Friday, July 29

I was on call Wednesday night and it was horrible. I've suddenly come to understand why some people say they don't like working at Jonas Bronck.

I was on call with the attending from hell. The night started with an argument, it ended with me accidentally giving the wrong dose of a medication that the patient didn't even need, and there was a whole lot of other ugly stuff that happened in between. The night was not fun, not fun at all.

The day started off quietly. I only had three patients, and I was getting ready to discharge one of them, a patient with RAD [Reactive Airway Disease, also known as asthma]. In the afternoon, before sending the kid home, I checked with Dr. Cintron, the attending who was on call with me that night. I presented the case to her quickly, telling her the kid had RAD.

She said, "Why do you say he has RAD? Why don't you say he has asthma?"

Now, I learned that RAD was the term you used for someone who was wheezing but didn't have a history strong enough to say it was a recurrent thing, which is what I learned asthma actually is. This child had had an episode of bronchiolitis [inflammation of the smaller airways of the lung caused by a viral infection that leads to wheezing; many children who have bronchiolitis in infancy go on to develop asthma when older] *a couple of months ago, but he hadn't been admitted. This was his first episode since then, and I didn't want to label him as being a full-blown asthmatic yet.*

"Well, that's what asthma is," Dr. Cintron told me. "RAD is just a cop-out. You've either got asthma or you don't."

Fine. Whatever she wanted to call it. It wasn't worth arguing about. The bottom line was that she agreed that we could send the child home.

So we got that kid out of the hospital. The night started and we got one admission after the other. Thank God we had a nurse practitioner on with us. Those nurse practitioners are great. They do the work of doctors and they're so nice. It's a pleasure having them around.

On Wednesday night, our nurse practitioner was a godsend, because sometime during the night, I developed a splitting headache. At 11:30, after being on my feet nonstop for eight straight hours, I had to finally stop, take a couple of aspirins, and sit down. Wouldn't you know, good old Dr. Cintron decided to choose just that moment to come into the nurses' station. She saw me sitting there and said, "Oh no, we can't have this. You can't sit down. If I'm standing, you're standing, too." I thought to myself, "Bless you, you asshole, bless you," but I held my tongue.

Anyway, around then, I got paged by the nurses to come look at a baby from one of the other teams in the PICU [Pediatric Intensive Care Unit]. *I'd never seen this baby before, but because of the way night call works at the Bronck, I wound up being responsible for him. He's a six-week-old who was admitted a couple of weeks ago with apnea* [literally, not breathing]. *As a newborn, he spent time in the NICU, was discharged at four weeks of age, and came back a few days later with apnea. Apparently, he was better last week, but in the last few days he's had an increase in his number of episodes. So I got a sign out that said to watch him closely.*

Before leaving that afternoon, his intern had done a blood gas [a test measuring the levels of oxygen, carbon dioxide, and acid in the blood], *which showed he was a little hypoxic* [had a low level of oxygen in his blood]. *The kid probably has some BPD* [bronchopulmonary dysplasia, a chronic lung disease not uncommon in premature babies]. *At least that was my assessment.*

Anyway, we went on rounds at about 1:00 A.M., and Cintron didn't think the kid's lungs sounded so good, so we gave him a stat Proventil treatment [an inhaled medication that dilates small airways] *and repeated the blood gas. He was still hypoxic, but slightly less so than before. I was sure this was his baseline and I wasn't concerned, but then Cintron came by and listened to his lungs again and said, "You know what? He sounds wet. Wet, wet, wet, wet, wet!" And I'm thinking, "Okay, lady, just get to the part where I'm supposed to care." She said she thought we should give him some Lasix* [a powerful diuretic used for lots of different purposes; in this case, it was being used in an attempt to decrease the amount of fluid in the baby's lungs].

I was looking at her thinking, "Give me a break, lady. It's three o'clock in the morning, the kid is doing fine, he ain't turning blue, he ain't having any apnea or respiratory distress. Why not just leave him the hell alone?" I finally expressed some of these senti-ments in slightly more polite terms, but Cintron disagreed with me. "No," she kept saying, "He needs Lasix. He sounds wet, wet, wet, wet, wet!"

God give me strength.

That's when I really started to hate this woman. Prior to this point, I had merely been irritated by her, but now I really had the urge to strangle her. Normally, I wouldn't give a damn, but giving Lasix to a baby this size isn't without risk. All we needed to do for this kid was dry him out in the middle of the night and totally screw up his electrolytes. I was taught that after 5:00 P.M., if something ain't broke, don't try to fix it. This baby was doing fine. Why not just leave him alone?

Why not leave him alone? Because this crazy attending had made up her mind, and once it was made up, there was apparently no changing it. Fine. I didn't argue. I wrote the order for Lasix. The nurse told me that since it was given by IV push, I'd have to give it myself. I told her fine, if she drew it up, I'd give it. At about this point, I snuck into the back of the PICU, shoved three chairs together, and lay down. I actually had the crazy notion that I was going to get some sleep back there.

Not! Ten minutes later, the Lasix was drawn up and the nurse came and handed it to me. I was groggy, but I went to the kid's bedside, flushed the IV with saline, pushed the Lasix, then flushed again with more saline. I was done in less than a minute.

Now, I probably should have gone back into the back of the PICU and tried to get some sleep, but I figured, what the hell, I'll take care of some of my scut work. So I was sitting at the computer looking up lab results when the PICU nurse runs up to me holding the order book [the looseleaf notebook in which the interns write all the nursing orders, including doses of medications, for the patients] *in her hands.*

Now, before I go any further, I should explain that in med school, I learned that when you write orders, you first write the name of the drug, then the concentration of the drug, then the dose you want to give. At the Bronck, though, they told me to write the dosage you want to give in milligrams per kilogram, and the nurse will figure it out herself. Well, that's what I was told to do, but apparently it's not true, because I wrote down the concentration of the drug, 10 milligrams per kilogram, and that's what the nurse gave me. This child was supposed to get a total of 1 milligram per kilogram; he wound up getting more than three times that dose. And that's not good.

Now, I wasn't alarmed. With an overdose of Lasix, all that happens is that instead of peeing out a little fluid, the kid would be expected to pee out a lot of fluid. We can take care of that: As long as we keep on top of it, all we have to do is give him back a little extra fluid through his IV. If we monitor the amount of urine he produces and make sure we replace it, we should have been able to all get through this.

But of course, that's not how Dr. Cintron figured it. She was hysterical. She came running in, screaming, "Oh no, how could you make such a mistake? We're going to have to write up an incident report, we're going to have to monitor him closely. Get another blood gas and a new set of lytes [electrolytes] right now!" And I'm thinking, "Oh Jesus, if we'd just left this kid alone, if she hadn't decided to mess with him in the middle of the night when there wasn't really anything wrong with him to begin with, none of this shit would've happened and we'd all be off sleeping now."

By that point, it was about 4:30. I'd been locked up in that PICU nearly all night long. Plus, on top of that, my headache had come back with a vengeance, and this damned pip-squeak of an attending wasn't doing anything to make my head feel any better. But I didn't say anything; I kept myself under control. I knew if I let myself go, I would have killed that girl, just strangled her by the neck until she was dead.

I drew the new blood gas, I sent it down to the lab, and, of *course, they called a few minutes later to tell me it was "QNS"* [quantity not sufficient]. *I wanted to tell them to QN my ass! But I didn't. I kept myself under control. And I had to repeat the whole damned thing.*

So I got the new sample, ran it down to the lab, and this time it ran fine. The gas was perfect. Of course, the bitch Cintron took a look at it and said, "Well, it's not great, but I guess it'll have to do." Bitch!

By this point, the sun was coming up. It had had the potential to be a great night, but because I was on with this witch, neither the baby nor I had anything resembling a good night. I hate this woman. I really hate her.

Erica Cintron wasn't the only attending with whom Denise had a run-in during her months at Jonas Bronck. On August 2, she made this entry:

Earlier in the day, I was trying to discharge a patient, a little boy who'd had head trauma. He'd spent two days in the hospital just being observed, and it had turned out that he was fine. In addition to his head trauma, he'd also had some belly trauma, and so they'd done a CAT scan of his abdomen in the ER before he'd been admitted. His belly had been fine by the time he'd reached the floor, and I'd never heard anything about the results of the CAT scan. So before he left, I figured I'd go track down the study.

I went down to the basement of the Bronck, where pediatric radiology is located. I started looking for the films, but I couldn't find them anywhere. It was as if they'd disappeared off the face of the Earth. I looked all over for them and neither I nor the X-ray tech could find them. Finally, they turned up in a really obvious place: in the radiologist's office, under his desk. Of course! Why hadn't I thought to look there first? Who the hell knows what they were doing down there? Anyway, the important thing was I finally had them, and I took them over to Dr. Silverberg, the radiologist, to have them read.

Jesus Christ, what a useless human being that man is! This man can never give you a straight answer. You show him an X ray and say, "Dr. Silverberg, does this patient have pneumonia?" and he says, "Well, it might be pneumonia, I certainly can't rule out pneumonia, but it also might be mucous plugging, or atelectasis, or maybe it's nothing at all. It could be completely normal." I swear, that man hedges so much that he should have weeds growing out of his ass.

And not only that, but every morning during X-ray rounds, which, I might point out, are totally useless, he gives us the same damned speech. "Why did you get this X ray? There was no need to get this X ray. You shouldn't have gotten this X ray." From med school, I'm used to people looking at X rays and saying, "This one's negative, this one shows pneumonia, this one shows a broken rib." I'm used to getting straight answers, not this "well, it might be this, but then again it might be that" crap. That man's so frustrating. I just can't take this shit.

Anyway, I gave him the films and told him the boy's story. I said I just wanted to make sure the study was normal before sending the kid home. That's all I wanted. But that's not all he wanted to tell me. What he wanted to do was give me a whole big lecture that it was my responsibility to follow up and why did I order this CAT scan if I wasn't planning on checking on it for two days? I wanted to say, "Look, pal, you are letting precious minutes slip away here, and I've got things to do. Just tell me if the films are normal or not."

Of course, the films were negative. But it took me nearly an hour to get this important information out of that man. What a waste! An absolute waste!

To me, it's amazing how two interns at the same level of training, working in the same residency program, can spend time with the same attending physician and come to exactly opposite conclusions about him. Although Denise Powers wasn't exactly in love with the teaching methods of Herb Silverberg, the pediatric radiologist at the Bronck, Hal Burkins was very much taken with the man. During November and December, while rotating through Jonas Bronck, Hal came into close contact with Dr. Silverberg. Near the end of his rotation, here's what Hal had to say about the radiologist:

Educationally, I've had an exceptionally good time at Jonas Bronck. The best part of it has been my interaction with Dr. Silverberg, the pediatric radiologist. He's really phenomenal. He comes up every day and shows us the X rays that were done the day before, and he beats on us and beats on us until he gets us thinking about things. For each film, Dr. Silverberg asks, "Why did you get this X ray? What questions did you want the X ray to answer?" So that rather than everything being automatic, just a knee-jerk response, we have to think through exactly why an X ray was ordered. He really guides us and makes us think and broaden our differential diagnosis for each of the different cases.

During the two months, we've had some really interesting cases that he's helped us through. We had a pulmonary sequestration [a congenital anomaly of the lung in which the blood supply to one or more lobes arises from an aberrant source], *we had a loculated pneumonia with pleural effusion, and an intussusception* [a condition in which one portion of the small intestine telescopes itself into the adjacent portion of the bowel, causing an obstruction; intussusception is dangerous, because it can cause the cutting off of the blood supply to that portion of the bowel, leading to necrosis, rupture, and a severe infection]. *He'd take all the X rays, go over the clinical features of the case, demonstrate the radiologic findings, and really put the whole thing together. It was fantastic; he really taught us a lot. I feel really fortunate to have had the opportunity to work with him.*

So Hal saw Dr. Silverberg as a superb teacher, a man who brought radiology to life, while Denise viewed him as a silly old man who accomplished little more than waste her time. Whose view is correct?

As has already been mentioned, the role of a residency training program is to prepare house officers to function as attending physicians. Although service to patients is a necessary part of the job, interns should get more out of interactions with attending physicians than simply the interpretation of an X ray, orders about what ventilator settings should be used for a premature infant, or instructions regarding where urinalyses should be performed. They need to understand why certain X-ray findings imply specific medical problems, what purpose is accomplished by using those ventilator settings, how that urinalysis should properly be performed. So from the point of view of what constitutes good teaching, I believe Hal's view of Dr. Silverberg's method is the correct one.

Dr. Silverberg's teaching skills and general usefulness were not the only subjects about which Denise and Hal disagreed. More and more on the pediatric service at Jonas Bronck, physician's assistants and pediatric nurse practitioners play an important role. Throughout her diary entries, Denise continually praises the PAs and PNPs; she loved the way they seemed to anticipate when life was becoming overwhelming for the interns and then, without hesitation, would pitch in and help by taking admissions, doing scut work, writing chart notes, or just plain being empathetic. At the end of August, as she finished her rotation, Denise's main regret about leaving the Bronck was that she was going over to the west campus where she wouldn't have PAs or PNPs to help her out.

This was not the conclusion reached by Hal Burkins. In his entry from Friday, October 28, here's what he had to say about PAs and PNPs:

The issue of having physician's assistants and nurse practitioners managing patients is kind of scary to me. These people don't have a strong background in physiology and pathology. Externally, we're all listening to the same symptoms and treating those symptoms, but the M.D.s have a broader and deeper understanding of the cause of the patient's illness and the care they need. In general, we see the patients when they're acutely ill, we follow them overnight and into the next day, and then we see them as they recover from their illness. That's a lot different from what the PAs do; they manage the patients' daily routines from eight to five, but they don't go much beyond that.

I'm not sure what the implications of this kind of system are for the future of medicine. Is the future going to call for PNPs and PAs to have greater roles in the management of patients? If they can prescribe medications and write orders, then what will the role of the physician be? It's a little scary to think about. It almost makes you want to go into a subspecialty so that you'll be assured of having a place in the medical system of the future. Will it become so fractionated that a new medical specialty will develop that only deals with the management of inpatients, doctors who never deal with an ambulatory patient? I'm not quite sure. But it does seem as if the days when a physician could take care of patients in an office and then take care of them when they're admitted to the hospital might be coming to an end. I'm not sure how any of this is going to work out.

So Denise saw PNPs and PAs as partners, colleagues, and comembers of the medical care delivery team, while Hal viewed these same individuals as competitors, vying for the same market share, forcing major changes in the future of his career. These two views, of both Dr. Silverberg's teaching style and of the role of physician's assistants, foreshadow how both Hal and Denise deal with future stresses during the course of this internship year.

3

SEPTEMBER

The Third Rotation:
Our Beloved Ancillary Staff

On the morning of the first day of the first clinical rotation of my third year of medical school, Matt Winston, the intern to whom I'd been assigned, took me aside and said to me: "Bob, I'm going to give you some important advice. If you want to make it through your training in one piece, there are two groups of people with whom you should never fight. The first are the lab technicians. The second are the elevator operators. If you get into a fight with a member of either of these two groups, you might as well start filling out applications to law school, because from that moment on, your life in medicine will be absolute misery."

Being impressionable, I listened to Matt's advice. As my own training evolved, I realized how accurate his words had been. I learned that no matter what you learn in medical school or what you come to believe from watching such informative TV shows as *ER*, it's not the doctors who run the hospital, it's the non-M.D.s. Nurses provide direct care to patients; lab techs determine how rapidly (or, actually, how slowly) tests are run. And at least at Jonas Bronck, elevator operators, the hospital employees with the absolute least amount of training in the entire system, determine how rapidly the doctors reach the floor during emergencies. Getting into an argument with even one of these staff members will translate into a year's worth of pain and torture.

The reason for this (not to sound overparanoid) is that members of these ancillary services tend to stick together. Argue with one lab technician, and you've essentially argued with every lab technician from each of the three shifts that make up a twenty-four-hour hospital day. Fight with an elevator operator, and you'll spend the rest of the year taking the fire stairs up eight flights to the ward.

So through my years of medical school, internship, and residency, I made it my business to follow Matt Winston's advice. Although I tried my best, there were clearly times when my nerves frayed. I nearly always managed to restrain myself, but there was one case in which I simply exploded.

That one case occurred on a Sunday during the middle of my senior residency year. I was tired, it had been a trying day on call, and I had a headache. I was spending that month working on the pediatric ward at University Hospital, and that afternoon we had admitted an unfortunate three-month-old baby who'd been transferred from Jefferson Hospital in the South Bronx. The infant, who'd been born twelve weeks prematurely to a heroin-addicted woman, had suffered an intracranial hemorrhage (a hemorrhage into the substance of the brain, a not unusual consequence of extreme prematurity) during his first few days of life. As a result of the hemorrhage, the baby developed hydrocephalus, a buildup of cerebrospinal fluid in the ventricular system of the brain. He'd come to us so that our neurosurgeon, Dr. Jeffrey Sheldon, could place a ventriculoperi-toneal shunt—a piece of plastic that would drain the excess fluid from his brain into his abdomen—into him.

The baby was scheduled for surgery the following morning. After arriving on the pediatric floor, he was taken into the treatment room where I, along with the pediatric intern who was on call that day and the medical student who was working with him, examined him. The child looked and acted pretty much the way I'd expected he would: tiny and wasted. His head looked way too big for his body, a result of the hydrocephalus. The kid had clearly suffered severe brain damage: He didn't smile, make eye contact, fix or follow objects, or respond at all to sounds. "Terrific," I said to the intern while we were examining him, "a real save! What a great job they're doing at Jefferson Hospital!"

While we were finishing with the baby, the neurosurgery resident on call poked his head through the treatment room's door. "Where's Dr. Sheldon's new patient?" he asked. Pissed-off, I didn't answer; I just glared at him and then looked down at the infant, whose beachball-sized head should have been a dead giveaway. "Is this him?" the guy eventually asked.

"Maybe," I replied. "What if it is?"

"I just want to make sure you know he's scheduled to go to the OR tomorrow at eight. Be sure to send off the pre-op bloods and make sure he's NPO [meaning that he should be given nothing by mouth] after midnight."

"Pre-op bloods? What do you mean?" I asked. I really was in a bad mood.

"You know, pre-op bloods," the resident replied, not sure what was going on. He knew I was a senior resident, and was trying to figure out whether I was pulling his leg or had suddenly developed Alzheimer's. "CBC [complete blood count], type and cross, the usual stuff we do before surgery."

"Oh, of course, we'll send those," I said. "I thought you meant something special."

Now really confused, the guy backed himself out of the treatment room and left. "Well, you heard the man," I told the intern and medical student. "Send off those pre-op bloods and make sure he's NPO after midnight. Any questions?"

The intern and medical student didn't have any, so, leaving them to get the scut done, I went back to the nurses' station and wrote my admission note.

About an hour later, I was still in the nurses' station when the intern came at me. "I can't get it," he said.

"Can't get what?" I asked.

"I can't get the pre-op bloods. I've stuck this kid at least ten times, and I haven't gotten a single drop out of him. The kid's aveinic [medicalese for 'having no veins']."

I sighed and slowly lifted myself from my seat. My headache had passed, but I was still really tired. The last thing I wanted to do was get blood out of a tiny premie who'd survived three months of the holocaust that is neonatal intensive care. I knew that after all he'd been through, this kid wasn't likely to have any veins or arteries that would yield a substantial amount of blood, but I also knew that if I didn't get it, Dr. Sheldon was going to spend most of the next morning kicking my butt around the hospital. With all this in mind, I followed the intern and medical student back into the treatment room.

The intern was right: That pitiful infant was totally aveinic. Before stabbing him with a twenty-three gauge-butterfly needle, I surveyed every square inch of his puny little body; I tied rubber band tourniquets around every limb; I placed the rubber band around the top of his head; I felt every pulse point for signs of an artery pumping away below the skin. Nowhere did I find anything that I would call a likely candidate to surrender enough of the fluid we needed to properly pre-op him. So, in the end, in desperation, I went for the blind stick.

Like the intern before me, I wound up sticking that poor baby again and again. Finally, just about the time I was beginning to accept the fact that I had failed, I stuck a needle under the skin of his left forefoot. Suddenly, the tubing attached to the butterfly needle filled with bright red blood. Pulling back on the syringe, I managed to suck out three cc's before the strike gave out. But three cc's was more than enough. I squirted one cc of the blood into a purple top tube for the CBC and the rest into a red top tube to be sent to the blood bank for the type and cross match, a test that would allow blood to be available in case the baby needed a transfusion during the course of the operation. "Make sure these make it down to the lab," I said, handing the tubes to the intern. As I passed through the door of the treatment room, I smiled as I heard the intern say, "Make sure these make it down to the lab," to the medical student.

It was after 9:00 P.M., and I was almost finished making night rounds with the ward's head nurse when the intern approached. "I just got a call from the blood bank. There's a problem with the type and cross on the new neurosurgical baby."

"What kind of a problem?" I asked, truly having no idea how anything could have gone wrong. "You guys hand-delivered the tube, didn't you?"

"Absolutely," he answered. "The medical student dropped it off himself. But apparently, he didn't sign and date it."

"Well, that's no problem," I replied. "Just go down there, get the specimen, sign it, date it, and hand it back to them."

"That's what I figured I'd do," the intern said. "But when I got down there and asked for it, the technician told me I couldn't have it. He said it had to be signed at the time it was drawn, and that since it wasn't, he was going to have to discard it."

"Discard it!" I roared, my anger flashing. "Did you tell him how hard it was to get that tube of blood? Did you mention how many times we had to stick that baby in order to get it?"

"I told him, but it didn't help," the intern replied. "He said we'd have to send down another tube if we wanted him to do the type and cross match."

"Let me speak to the guy." I walked to the nurses' station and called the blood bank's number. When the technician picked up, in my sweetest, nicest, talking-to-a-lab-technician voice, I said, "Hi, this is Bob Marion; I'm the senior resident on pediatrics tonight. My intern told me that there was some problem with the type and cross on a baby we sent down earlier this evening?"

"No, no problem," the man replied. "The tube wasn't signed, so I discarded it. I need another sample, signed by the doctor who drew it, if you want blood available for surgery."

"Look, I know you guys require that the tube be signed at the time it's drawn, and I understand that you do that to protect the patient against the possibility of a mix-up that could lead to a transfusion reaction, but this is a special case. This is a very small, very sick premature baby. We had to stick him about twenty times to get that blood. Couldn't you make an exception just this once and give us the tube back? I drew the blood myself, and I'll guarantee that it's this baby's blood."

"If you had such a hard time drawing it, doctor, you should have been more careful in handling it," the guy responded to my impassioned plea. "I'm sorry, but I have no choice. My directions are to discard any tube that arrives here unsigned."

My anger was beginning to rise. "I know you have rules, and I also know that exceptions can sometimes be made. Is there someone else I could speak to about this? Your supervisor or someone?"

"You can speak to anyone you like," the technician said, "but it isn't going to make any difference. I've already discarded the tube. If you want the type and cross done, you'd better get me another tube."

And with those words, he hung up.

By hanging up the phone, that lab tech managed to push me over the precipice I'd managed to avoid passing over since the start of my medical training. I had started the day tired, and now I was pissed off. I wasn't going to let a blood bank tech hang up on me, a senior resident in charge of the entire pediatric service. I was going to go down there and get that tube of blood even if I had to wrestle the guy for it. I was going to get the tube, sign it right in front of him, and if he refused to do the type and cross, I was going to report him to the union, the hospital's administrator-on-duty, the medical director, and the president of the whole medical center. This jerk had chosen the wrong guy to mess with!

Running down the stairs, taking them two and three at a time, I made it to the third floor in record time. Striding into the blood bank, I found my adversary hard at work at a lab bench. "Can I help you?" he asked sweetly.

"No, thanks," I replied. "You've done enough already." Without another word, I found the lab's garbage barrel and began emptying it, piece of trash by piece of trash, onto the floor.

"Hey, what the hell are you doing?" he asked, growing concerned. After all, it was late, he was alone in the lab, and his world had been invaded by an apparent madman who was angrily sifting through the trash.

"I'm looking for that sample you threw out," I screamed.

"You may not give a shit about how much pain we had to put that baby through in order to get this sample, but I sure as hell do."

"Get out of here," the guy yelled, backing up toward the lab's door and holding an Erlenmeyer flask in his left hand, apparently for protection. "Get out of here right now, or I'll call security."

"I'm not leaving until I get that fucking specimen," I yelled back at him, certainly not intimidated by his threats. "Just tell me where that tube is and I'll leave you alone."

"I told you on the phone, I discarded it," the guy yelled.

"Where?" I yelled back again. "Where did you discard it?"

"I poured the blood down the sink."

"What?" I screamed. "You poured the blood down the sink. What kind of an idiotic asshole are you?"

"Those are my instructions," the guy replied. "If a specimen comes in unsigned, we are told to pour the tube's contents down the sink and call the doctor to inform him."

By this point, the yelling had attracted technicians from the other labs down the hall. They stood out in the hall, a safe enough distance away so that no debris that might come flying out of the lab could hit them. I saw them out there and knew that I was making a scene, but I just couldn't control myself anymore.

"Do you realize what you've done? Do you have any idea how hard it's going to be to get another specimen from that baby? Would you like to come up to the ward and try to get blood out of this kid? Or better yet, how about if I stick you with a needle fifteen or twenty times, just so you can understand how stupid your fucking rule is? Would you like that, having a needle stuck into you fifteen or twenty times?"

Before he could respond, a hospital security guard entered

the lab. "What's going on?" he asked, immediately coming between the technician and me.

"This jackass discarded a specimen on a baby who's impossible to get blood from," I said. The sudden appearance of the guard helped me get my anger back under control.

"He just ran in here and started attacking me," the technician said.

"Physically attacking you?" the guard asked. "Did he hit you?"

"No," the technician replied, "verbally attacked me. But I wouldn't put physical violence past him. He's a very menacing person."

"Look, Doc," the guard said, "you'd better go back to wherever it is you belong. I don't care what happened here, but I don't want any more of this behavior. And I don't think it would be such a good idea for you to come back down to these labs tonight." And then to both of us, he added: "I'm going to hang around here for a while. I don't want any trouble. Do you understand?"

I nodded and walked out of the blood bank. Taking the elevator back up to the pediatric ward without saying a word to anyone, I picked the baby up out of his crib, carried him into the treatment room, and began to stick him again. This time, I managed to get the sample on the fourth stick. He didn't respond much to the sticking; he was neurologically too far gone to feel much. After I'd managed to fill up the tube, I signed it and handed it to the intern. He did what had to be done, and I went off to sleep.

The next morning at precisely eight o'clock, the baby was in the operating room. The surgery went wonderfully. In the blood bank, two units of blood had been matched to the sample the intern had brought down the night before. The procedure was uncomplicated and no bleeding occurred; the units of blood were never needed.

During the last few months of my residency, I never again set foot on the third floor of University Hospital. And even now, when I have to go to the laboratory area for a meeting, I nervously look both ways, worried that I might run into that blood bank technician.

It was in September that the little things like relationships with members of affiliated services began to get to the interns. September is when the little inconveniences of being an intern begin to take their toll: the "specialness" has worn off (usually, the specialness wears off by about the middle of July), the exhaustion caused by spending too many hours in the hospital begins to exert its effect, and there's not even a hint that the end is in sight. So take a stressed, overtired intern, add the fact that, in order to get his work done, he has to interact with members of an array of services whose tasks and goals don't coincide with his, and you can understand how friction can occur. This is the recipe that in September of 1994 led to the doctor's orders war between Scott Lindsay and the nurses on the children's unit at Mt. Scopus.

To be honest, the doctor's orders war in September wasn't the first skirmish Scott had with the nursing staff. His troubles began back in August. In his diary entry of August 18, he describes a terrible night on call during which he spent more than thirty-three consecutive hours awake and working on Six-A, the general pediatric ward at West Bronx Hospital. This is how the night ended:

To top it off, I'd been in the hospital since 7:00 yesterday morning, and today at 4:15 P.M., I was just finishing my sign out. I had written all the doctor's orders myself, and all of the sudden, this nurse came up to me and said, "Oh, Dr. Lindsay, can you rewrite this order?" She pointed in the order book to a prescription for Tylenol I'd written for a patient who'd come back from the operating room a few hours earlier where he'd had his tonsils removed. It was a routine order we always write on post-op patients. The idea is that if the kid develops a fever or complains of pain, the nurses won't hassle us in the middle of the night for a Tylenol order.

I looked at the order and it looked perfectly fine to me, so I asked, "Why do you want it rewritten?" She told me it was because I'd written over the "T" in Tylenol a few times, and it wasn't completely clear. I said, "It looks clear to me." She said the head nurse had told her not to pick up the order unless it's made clearer. I said, "Sorry, it looks fine to me. I'm not rewriting it."

Then the nurse said, "Well, I'm not giving the medication unless you rewrite it. And in fact, I can't make out most of the rest of these orders. If you don't rewrite all of them, I'm not going to be able to pick up any of them."

I started to get really pissed. I said, "Look, this is my handwriting. I may not have the best handwriting, but it is clearly legible." And then I pointed to the order for IV fluids and said, "What does this say?" She read it perfectly: "D5 1/2 normal saline with 20 milliequivalents of potassium chloride per liter at twenty cc's per hour. But it doesn't matter. The nursing supervisor won't allow me to pick up these orders unless they're written more clearly. If I pick them up, I could get cited."

I felt like saying, "Piss off, bitch." Even though it would have taken me no more than seconds to rewrite the orders, it was the principle. I mean, it wasn't like I scribbled the orders in Chinese or some other obscure language. They were written in perfectly understandable English and, although I'll be the first to admit that I don't have the greatest handwriting, every person she asked could easily read them. And there was just no way, after being in the hospital for so long, that I was going to rewrite those orders just to make that goddamned bitch happy.

I would have taken on the nursing supervisor and the hospital administrator and anyone else they wanted to throw at me, but fortunately it didn't go any further. My resident, who'd been watching this whole thing from across the nurses' station, finally got off her butt and did something about it. She came over and said to the nurse, "Look, he's tired, just leave him alone," and she volunteered to rewrite the orders for me. The nurse shrugged, said something like, "As long as somebody rewrites them, I don't care who does it," and walked away, looking for someone else whose life she could make miserable.

When she was gone, I said to my resident, who was copying over my perfectly legible orders, "Marge, this whole thing is one big LOS!"

She asked me what LOS meant and I told her, "LOS means Load of Shit." She looked around and said, "Scott, you've got to watch what you say. There are parents all over the place." I realized there were parents around and I do have to watch some of the things that come out of my mouth, but I just couldn't help it: I was tired and this nurse just keeps me perpetually pissed off!

Scott made it through the rest of August without any more trouble, but it was his difficulty with penmanship that led to the doctor's orders war that occurred on the children's unit in September.

Working on the children's unit at Mt. Scopus is not exactly a piece of cake. Many of the children on the ward have cancer and some are terminally ill; others have neurologic diseases, like severe cerebral palsy, that have reduced them to a vegetative state; still others have chronic diseases that cause them to develop more and more medical problems over time. For interns, dealing with these children and their families can be a stressful experience.

Although Children's is stressful, one thing that makes life easier is the terrific nursing staff. But Scott Lindsay's life wasn't made easier. And as the attending physician assigned to that unit that month, I not only got to observe the situation, I was privileged to serve as an active participant.

Before getting into the story of the doctor's orders war, I should explain what they are: The orders are the instructions from the medical staff to the nursing staff that spell out the patient's exact method of care. Early in medical school, we're taught the proper form for writing orders, and during the third and fourth years of med school, with the guidance of interns and residents, we gain enough experience to become expert at the task. So unchanging are the orders that by the time September of internship has rolled around, the interns can pretty much write orders in their sleep (which often is not far from the state in which they are actually written).

The orders follow a standard form. They are remembered by young and old doctors alike by the mnemonic ABC-DAVID. These letters stand for:

1. *Admit to* (whatever ward to which the patient is being admitted).

2. *Because of* (the diagnosis is listed on this line).

3. *Condition* (this is the line from which the media gets the information that a patient is in "critical" condition; in most hospitals, it is standard that any patient admitted to an intensive care unit is listed as being in critical condition).

4.   Diet (wherein the food the patient is allowed to eat is noted; for patients who are scheduled for surgery or who, for other reasons, are not allowed food by mouth, the letters "NPO" are listed here).

5.   Activity (whether the patient must remain in bed or is allowed to get up and roam around).

6.   Vital signs (that is, how often the patient's pulse and respiratory rates, blood pressure, and temperature should be monitored by the nursing staff).

7.   Intake and output (that is, whether the nursing staff should keep track of how much the patient eats and gets through the IV, and how much urine, stool, and vomitus is lost).

8.   Drugs (in these last lines, the medications, their doses, and the frequency with which they're to be given are listed; also noted here are orders for the intravenous fluids, including the concentration of electrolytes and rate at which it should drip through the tubing and into the vein).

Early in their careers, interns learn that hidden within the bare bones of these orders lie a multitude of opportunities to torture the nursing staff. For instance, ordering that a patient's intake and output be strictly monitored and that every ounce of urine produced be scrupulously collected can add hours of horrendously unpleasant work to the nurses' already overloaded list of tasks.

Scott Lindsay's month on Children's began innocently enough. The floor was running at about two-thirds capacity, and on the Wednesday morning on which the rotation began, Scott picked up only three patients: a four-year-old boy with leukemia who'd been admitted the day before for his regularly scheduled course of chemotherapy; a nine-year-old girl with osteogenic sarcoma [a malignant tumor of the bone] whose Hickman line [a permanent indwelling catheter that allows medications and IV fluids to be given without the need for starting a new IV] had become infected and now required three weeks of intravenous antibiotics in order to clear the infection; and an eight-year-old boy with Joubert syndrome, a rare neurodegenerative disease that had left the child severely impaired, who had developed pneumonia and was receiving oxygen and antibiotics. In his first hours on the ward, Scott spent his time reviewing these patients' charts, introducing himself to the children and their parents, and informing them that he was now going to be their doctor.

Problems didn't begin until the following Tuesday. On the children's unit, Tuesday is order renewal day. At noon every Tuesday, all standing orders on every patient become null and void. In the morning, the interns are required to rewrite every order on every patient, essentially forcing them to readmit each child on their service.

On the first Tuesday of his rotation on Children's, Scott was not exactly in a terrific mood. Having been on call on Monday, he'd had a bad night and gotten no sleep. During the previous twenty-four hours, he'd admitted six new patients, two of whom, becoming sicker after admission, had wound up transferred to the intensive care unit. On top of that, the week before he'd developed an intestinal virus that had blossomed over the weekend. As a result, over the last few nights, he'd spent more time in the bathroom than he had in bed. Scott was not in the best shape.

And, of course, his handwriting reflected this condition. Worse than usual, his orders were now nearly incomprehensible. Not unexpectedly, Scott was called out of attending rounds, which had begun only minutes before, at a little after ten. What happened in the next few minutes are best detailed in a diary entry Scott recorded that Thursday:

When I reached the ward after leaving attending rounds, my friend Michelle [a nurse who'd been claiming she couldn't read his handwriting all month long] *was waiting for me at the nurses' station. "Dr. Lindsay," she said with an attitude, "I can't read these orders. Is this dose of Cefuroxime* [an antibiotic] *supposed to be 250 milligrams or 280 milligrams? Do you want it given every six hours or every eight? I can't read any of this stuff."*

I looked at the order. I'll admit it wasn't my best handwriting, but it clearly said "250 milligrams every six hours." I told her I thought it was pretty clear. "Well, I'm not picking it up unless you write it more legibly."

I figured it wasn't worth fighting about. So I sat down to write it again, doing it as neatly as I could. When I was done, I handed the order book back to her and asked if she could read it now. "Yeah, that one's fine," she said, "but the others are still unreadable. You have to rewrite all of them like that."

That's when I nearly lost it. I told her, "I'm not rewriting all these orders. Renewing orders is a waste of time in the first place. You know what all the orders are for all these patients, so rewriting them is just a technicality. I was up all night, I'm tired, and I have better things to do than waste my time rewriting these orders. I'm just not doing it."

She sneered at me and said, "Fine. If you don't rewrite them, I'm not going to pick them up."

I said, "Fine, don't pick them up. You do what you have to do and I'll do what I have to do. If this patient doesn't get what I've ordered, I'm going to report you to the chief of service. So do whatever the fuck you want."

I knew I shouldn't have said "fuck" out there in the nurses' station, but I wasn't feeling well, I was dead tired, and I didn't want to be dealing with all that just then. Anyway, Pat, the head nurse, who hadn't heard our conversation but had walked into the nurses' station right before I said "fuck," came up to me and literally pulled me by the shirt into the nurses' lounge. "Listen," she said, "I don't know much about you, and I don't know what your beef has been with Michelle, but don't you dare ever swear on my unit. I don't allow the patients or their families to do it, I'd kill any of my nurses if they were to do it, and I will not tolerate a doctor doing it."

I apologized and promised I'd try to prevent it from happening again, but I explained that I wasn't feeling well and that Michelle was torturing me about my handwriting for no reason at all. She was nice about it; she told me to go back to attending rounds and that she'd check into it.

Anyway, I was back in attending rounds no more than ten minutes when my pager went off again. Bob Marion, who's our attending this month, was getting a little annoyed. I mean, I was supposed to be presenting all the kids I'd admitted the night before and here I was, constantly getting paged out of rounds.

This time, it was Pat who paged me. She was waiting for me at the nurses' station. She said, "I looked over all the orders you wrote this morning and I agree with Michelle. Your handwriting is terrible. I'm not going to put any of my nurses in jeopardy by allowing them to pick them up. You have to rewrite each and every one of them."

I was so angry, I was speechless. I turned and walked back into the conference room. Bob saw how upset I was and asked what was wrong. I told him what had happened, and he said, "That's not right." Then he and Phil, our resident, came out to the nurses' station with me. Pat showed Bob the order book, and he came back to me and said, "I agree with Pat. These all have to be rewritten, but you're in no condition to do it. So after rounds, we'll each take one or two of your patients and rewrite all the orders."

That's how that problem was solved. After rounds, I went home and the rest of the team rewrote my orders. I've felt horrible about the whole thing since then. And I've been thinking about it a lot. I think I've figured out a way to get the nurses off my back.

When instituted during his next night on call, Scott's plan nearly got him permanently booted out of the hospital. Here's the account from his diary, recorded the next weekend:

The first patient I admitted on Friday afternoon was a ten-year-old with non-Hodgkins lymphoma who was coming into the hospital for a weekend of chemotherapy. Usually, the chemo kids come in during the week, but this girl's parents are trying to keep her life as normal as possible, and they've gotten the oncologists to admit her over the weekend so she doesn't miss school. Anyway, Dr. Goodwin, the oncologist, came by, gave me the girl's chemotherapy protocol, and told me to write the orders exactly as laid out in the protocol.

It turned out that Michelle was going to be this kid's nurse, so naturally, after I'd examined her, written my admission note and the doctor's orders, I got paged to the nurses' station. I called and Michelle got on the phone. "Guess what," she said, in that obnoxious voice of hers, "I can't read your orders. You're going to have to come back and rewrite them."

I asked her if she was sure she couldn't read them. She, of course, said she was sure. I said that the kid's protocol was in her chart. Would she maybe take a look at the protocol and follow the orders as written out in it? She told me she couldn't do that, that she had to get her orders directly from the doctor's orders sheets, and that I'd have to come back and rewrite them. I told her I'd be right there.

Look, you can't say I didn't give her a chance. It was clear that she was just doing this to torture me, that she was just trying to make my life miserable. If she'd just said "Yeah, okay, I'll just follow the protocol, no sweat," we would have had a nice night on call and nothing further would have happened. But no, she couldn't do that. So I did what I had to do.

What Scott had to do was rewrite the orders as neatly as possible, spelling out the name of each medication, its dose, and the frequency with which it was to be given in his very best handwriting. But in addition to this, in the same neat penmanship, he added the following order: Vital signs q 10 minutes.

Yes, he ordered Michelle to monitor the girl's respiratory and heart rates, her blood pressure and her temperature every ten minutes. Since it takes most of ten minutes for the vital signs to be properly checked and charted, if the orders were to be followed to the letter, Michelle and the nurses who followed her in the shifts to come would have to spend every minute of their time standing at this patient's bedside, endlessly monitoring her vital signs, enabling them to provide virtually no care to any other patient.

After finishing the orders, Scott took a seat at the nurses' station and, wearing a big smile, waited to see what would happen. He watched as Michelle picked up the order book, opened it to the page on which Scott's patient's orders were written, and, after muttering, "That's better," began copying out the orders onto the patient's cardex (the flip file on which a summary of the nursing assignment for each patient is listed). But when she got to the line about vital signs, Michelle stopped and looked up at the intern. "Are you having trouble reading them?" Scott asked, innocently.

"No, they're clear enough," she replied. "But I think you might have made a mistake here. You wrote for q 10 minute vital signs. You don't mean that, do you?"

"Of course I mean it," Scott replied. "The chemotherapy this patient is scheduled to receive is very toxic. The protocol says that vital signs must be frequently monitored."

"But every ten minutes is crazy. Wouldn't every hour be okay?"

"No, I want them done every ten minutes. That's what I wrote and that's what I want."

Michelle sighed, made another note in the cardex, and then put her pen down. "You're only doing this because of the problem with your handwriting. Q ten minute vital signs is crazy."

"It may be crazy, but that's what I've ordered. And as I understand it, you have to follow the orders."

And so, this battle in the ongoing war escalated. Michelle called Pat, who looked at the notation in the order book and said, "We can't do every ten minute vital signs."

"I want it done," Scott replied. "It says in the protocol that vital signs must be closely monitored. It's in the best interest of the patient and that's all that's important to me."

"It's ridiculous," Pat replied. "Why don't you just change it to every hour and we'll all forget the whole thing."

"I'm not forgetting anything. I want every ten minute vital signs and that's all there is to it."

"Scott, if you don't change it, I'm calling Dr. Logan." [Ned Logan is the chief of the pediatric service at Mt. Scopus.]

"Call Dr. Logan," Scott replied, glancing down at his watch. "I don't care who you call. All I know is, we've been arguing about this for so long, I think the vital signs are probably already overdue."

Within ten minutes, Ned Logan, two pediatric chief residents, the hospital's nursing supervisor, and I (in my role as attending physician for the month) had joined the parties already assembled in the nurses' station. Representing Michelle, Pat gave the nurses' side of the story. Scott, giving his side of the story, cited, among other items, the discriminatory treatment he'd received because he was "handwriting-impaired" (his term).

After hearing the evidence, it didn't take Ned Logan long to hand down a decision. "Scott, you will rewrite the vital sign order to read 'Vital signs every hour.' For the remainder of the month, you will also make every effort to write more clearly. Do you understand?"

Scott Lindsay reluctantly nodded his head.

"And although I sympathize with the nurses and understand that being sure of dose and timing of medications is important, it does appear that Scott has been discriminated against because of a problem over which he has little control. Pat, would you please have your nurses try to be more understanding with Scott for the rest of the month?"

The head nurse also nodded her head.

That was pretty much the end of it. During the last few weeks of that month, Scott did have to rewrite a few orders, but the harassment he'd been feeling abated significantly. No more fights occurred. At the end of September, Scott left the children's ward pretty much intact. Unfortunately, he carried with him more than just a month's worth of experience caring for patients: He now had a reputation among the nurses as a troublemaker. And as Matt Winston had told me nearly twenty years before, having a reputation like that can go a long way to making your life in medicine miserable.

4

OCTOBER

The Fourth Rotation: Res-Speak, a Guide to the Residency Subculture

One night in the middle of October 1979, I found myself fading. It was about 2:00 in the morning, I was working on Children's Five, the general pediatric ward at the Boston Medical Center, and I had just gotten an admission, an eighteen-month-old with asthma. I knew that if I put my mind to it, I could get everything done—including taking a history, doing a physical, starting an IV, writing orders, and giving medication and oxygen to stabilize the kid—in less than an hour. The problem was, I was so tired I was having trouble staying focused. What I needed to get me back on track was a hot cup of freshly brewed coffee.

Unfortunately, getting any kind of coffee at 2:00 A.M. at the Boston Medical Center was not an easy task. The hospital's snack bar and cafeteria were long closed by that hour, and although there were large pots set up in the nurses' lounges on each of the wards, coffee was only brewed in the early morning. After midnight, there might be a little something left in the bottom of the pot, but it wasn't exactly what you'd call drinkable.

That night, though, I was desperate, so I figured I'd give it a shot. And I lucked out: Jiggling the pot in the nurses' lounge on Children's Five, I knew there was some liquid down in there. By tipping and angling it, I managed to drain out about three-quarters of a cup. Having sat in that pot for at least twenty hours, the stuff was thick and bitter and nearly lethal. Although I prefer my coffee black, in order to get this stuff to a tolerable state, it was going to need a hell of a lot of milk and sugar.

I found the sugar without a problem, but there seemed to be no milk around anywhere. I looked in the refrigerator in the nurses' lounge and the patient refrigerator in the ward's pantry, but there was not a drop to be found. I tasted the coffee; no, the sugar wasn't going to be enough.

That's when I remembered that this, after all, was a pediatric ward, and although pediatric wards might not always have fresh milk, there had to be a plentiful supply of infant formula. Reaching into the floor's formula closet, I pulled out a four-ounce bottle of premixed Enfamil. I poured about an ounce of the formula into my Styrofoam coffee cup and, holding my nose, guzzled the mixture down. Within minutes, the caffeine rush exploded through my body. With this artificial burst of energy, I got back to work. By 3:15, that asthmatic and I were both lying in our respective beds, breathing comfortably and snoring away.

Although that mixture worked its magic that night, I realized almost immediately that by drinking that rancid coffee laced with Enfamil, I'd crossed a line, descending into a deeper level of housestaff hell. Day-old coffee lightened with Enfamil is a beverage only a desperate intern would drink in the middle of the night. Downing that cup of coffee was yet another initiation into residency.

•

Because of the nature of their work, the lives led by interns and residents are very different from those of people not involved in medical training. Spending every third or fourth night in the hospital dealing with sick and dying patients, getting little or no sleep, and having virtually no free time does things to you, makes you live differently than other people.

As a result, interns and residents eat different food, sleep different hours, wear different clothes, socialize in different ways, even speak a different language from most normal people. Encountering an intern, especially one who is post-call, can be a disturbing experience.

The first book to really offer a glimpse of the residency subculture was Samuel Shem's *The House of God*. Because it portrayed the life as those of us in medicine actually knew it, *The House of God* became a cult classic, achieving immense success with medical students, interns, and residents.

Looking back on the book, published in the mid-seventies, it's amazing how out-of-date it now is. Back in the seventies, patients were routinely admitted to the hospital for elective evaluations, spending long, leisurely stays on the wards undergoing such procedures as "the bowel run of the stars" for days and days at a time. Of course, in the Golden Age of Managed Care, which is guided by the DRGs (*Diagnosis-Related Groups*—rules about how much reimbursement a hospital may receive for a specific diagnosis), not only would permission to admit a patient to the hospital for "the bowel run of the stars" be immediately denied, but the physician attempting to do so would be cited and ridiculed by his or her employer.

One part of *The House of God*, though, still rings true: the portrayal of some aspects of the lives led by the housestaff. This chapter, attempting to update some of the information contained in that book, is designed to help understand what makes house officers tick.

Part 1: The House Officer's Diet

Not surprisingly, my desperate search for coffee during that early October morning in 1979 was not an unusual occurrence. Working thirty-six hours straight means that sooner or later, you're going to have to eat a meal in the hospital. There are two problems with this: first, the timing of those meals; second, the meal's content.

It's usually not possible to take a lunch break at noon and knock off for dinner at 6:00 or 7:00 P.M. Interns and residents eat whenever and wherever they get the chance. Although the timing may coincide with what is usually considered normal mealtime, this is usually not the case.

During my years of training, the healthiest approach to eating I encountered was practiced by surgeons. During my third-year rotation in surgery, our team would meet in the cafeteria at Mt. Scopus Medical Center every morning at 6:00 A.M. The first morning of that rotation, I went through the line and grabbed my usual breakfast, a cup of black coffee and a bagel. "What's wrong?" our team's senior resident asked when I got back to the table. "You sick or something?" I explained I wasn't a big breakfast eater. He told me I'd better change my ways, or there was no way I'd ever make it through the clerkship. "This may be the only meal you get today," he said. "You'd better load up."

That's how the surgery housestaff approached life. The interns and residents piled the food on their cafeteria trays during breakfast: eggs and bacon, pancakes, French toast, bagels, donuts, and on and on, one plate piled on top of the other. And then they'd sit silently, polishing off every last morsel of food. When everyone was finished, they'd head for the operating room, where they might be called on to stand, scrubbed and concentrating, for ten or twelve hours without a break. After that breakfast, they would eat whenever they got the chance, but they would never be hungry.

We in pediatrics don't approach meals the way surgeons do, and, as a result, pediatricians wind up spending most of their days and nights starving, searching for something to eat. During on-call nights, food is usually ordered from neighborhood restaurants that deliver. Generally, at least in the Bronx, these restaurants are not the ones listed in the *Michelin Guide*. Usually, the food that arrives is tasteless, cold, and a nutritional nightmare.

The manner in which residents eat their meals is also unusual. I remember the meals I ate while working in the emergency room at Jonas Bronck. The only restaurant that would deliver was a bad Chinese take-out place located about a mile from the hospital. The food would be delivered and, between patients, each of us would run to the nurses' lounge to gobble it down. Since meals were served communal-style, we'd pour wonton soup into urine cups and the main course into plastic emesis basins (previously unused, of course). We'd use tongue depressors as utensils. The amazing thing was that none of us looked on any of this as unusual.

Hunger is always worst in the middle of the night. In most parts of the civilized world, it's difficult to find a restaurant that will deliver to a hospital ward at 2:00 or 3:00 in the morning. As a result, house officers spend a fair amount of time in the middle of the night foraging and scavenging for food. Desperate and starving at these hours, interns will eat just about anything.

Personally, I've eaten jars of baby food (some of my co-residents actually learned to love this stuff and would steal jars, especially the desserts, and take them home, to be consumed during their off nights), "renal cookies" (low sodium cookies intended for consumption by patients with renal failure; renal cookies are foul-smelling and foul-tasting, but if you're hungry enough, you'll eat them), and leftovers from patients' dinner trays. I'm sorry to say that on more than one occasion, I've even stolen candy from patients' personal stashes.

These disgusting dietary habits are not limited to meals eaten in the hospital, either. House officers not only don't cook, they barely even have time to see the inside of a grocery store.

Early in my internship, I developed a regular routine. Every post-call night on my way home from work, I stopped at the Watertown Pizza House ("You've tried the rest, now try the best!") and got a small pizza with extra cheese. I'd take it home, take off all of my clothes, climb into bed (after that bed was finally delivered by United Van Lines), and eat every last ounce of the pizza while watching reruns of *The Odd Couple*. Following the end of the show (which usually coincided with the end of the pizza), I'd pile the pizza box on top of all the other pizza boxes on my night table, turn off the TV, and fall asleep.

This approach to post-call eating has not changed in the years since the completion of my training. Here's a portion of Denise Powers's diary entry from July 12:

I stopped by the market on my way home from work, on account of the fact that I don't have any food in the house. So there I was, starving, tired, at the end of my rope, tripping through the aisles of the supermarket trying to find the things I needed.

It's really weird shopping for one person. I've never had to do it before. I got what I needed and, since it was late and I was so hun-

gry, I didn't want to come home and cook. So I got some fast food, which is probably going to send my cholesterol through the roof. Just what I need. But I don't care right now. I was hungry and I had to eat something.

This entry, made just two weeks after she'd begun her internship, started Denise on the downward slide that characterizes most house officers' dietary habits. Within weeks of this entry, she gave up all semblance of trying to keep food in her apartment. She, like so many others of us, wound up spending the rest of the year living on fast food.

Part 2: The House Officer Lifestyle

As mentioned in previous chapters, the house officer's main goal in life is to try to get sleep. Since the on-call schedule determines where and when sleep is most likely to occur, the intern's life pretty much revolves around this document.

During on-call mornings, the intern will awaken at about 6:00 A.M. and get ready for work. Getting dressed, he's likely to put on a soft, pajama-like scrub suit. These outfits, originally designed to be worn by surgeons in an attempt to maintain sterile technique in the operating room, have been co-opted by house officers from every specialty throughout the world for three major reasons:

1. They're amazingly comfortable.
2. They immediately let people know you're a doctor.
3. They make you look cool.

Scrub suits as on-call wear is a relatively recent phenomenon. Until the 1970s, most hospitals had a strict dress code for house officers, and except for time spent in the operating room, scrub suits were not part of that code. In the old days, on all wards and in every clinic and emergency room, doctors were required to wear hospital whites: white pants (or skirts for women), white shirts (with black ties), and white coats. In many hospitals, the system was so well enforced and pervasive that the only way to determine the seniority of a particular doctor was to check the length of the white coat he or she was wearing: If the white coat was very short, the doctor wearing it was an intern; if the coat was of intermediate length, the wearer was a resident; and if the coat came down to the knees or beyond, the person in it was an attending physician (or a butcher who had wandered in off the street).

But between Samuel Shem's *The House of God* in the mid-seventies and the start of my own internship in 1979, hospital whites became an optional component of house-officer fashion. And, at least in pediatrics, hospital whites were quickly eclipsed by the far more fashionable scrub-suit green.

In the old days, hospital whites were distributed to house officers. You'd pick them up at the hospital laundry, wear them until they were creased, covered with blood stains, and stank, and then traded them in for a clean set. All expenses were borne by the hospital.

The system with scrub suits, however, is not so well designed. Since they are technically forbidden to anyone other than surgeons, it is necessary for house officers from other specialties to "borrow" them from the surgery suite's locker room. Because they're compressible and easily hidden, this task is not difficult to accomplish. During my own internship, I managed to accumulate more than fifty sets of scrub suits from the locker room at the Boston Medical Center. I still have most of these scrubs and, to this day, still wear them as pajamas.

The wearing of a scrub suit in a hospital immediately identifies you as a house officer. During a senior residency rotation at University Hospital, one of my patients was Irwin, a nineteen-year-old man with Down syndrome who spent more than a month on the ward being treated for acute renal failure. Although short, Irwin was obese and didn't fit into any of the child-sized pajamas that were available on the floor. Unfazed, the nurses laid in a supply of scrub suits for Irwin.

Irwin loved wearing those scrub suits. During his time on the ward, he also developed something of a love affair with medicine. He would accompany us on work rounds every morning. He fit right in, tagging along with the group of house officers, medical students, and nurses, remaining quiet as we discussed each patient. One of the nurses gave him a broken stethoscope, and, like the rest of us, he'd drape it around his neck. Occasionally, we'd involve him in discussions: "Well, Doctor Irwin," one of us would say, "what do you think of the results of this SMA–6?" He'd always laugh and say, "I think he needs an operation."

A friendly and cooperative patient during the day, Irwin would become disoriented in the evening, a not unusual occurrence for hospitalized adults with Down syndrome. At least once a night, the nurses would find him wandering the corridor; they'd lead him back into his room, help him back into bed, and wait until he fell asleep again.

One night, though, Irwin wandered off the pediatric ward. After awakening, he threw his stethoscope around his neck as usual and headed into the hall, where he found the door to the stairwell open. Taking the stairs down two flights, he wound up wandering into the corridor of an internal medicine floor. When he reached the nurses' station, a nurse looked up and said, "Oh, doctor, I just paged you. I'm glad you got here so quickly. I'm worried about Mrs. Jones in 507. She's having some kind of arrhythmia [a disturbance in the rhythm of the heart]." The nurse handed Irwin a strip of EKG paper and began to lead him into Mrs. Jones's room. Irwin, who had seen us study EKGs on the pediatric ward, looked intensely at the squiggles on the long, thin strip of paper. Standing by the woman's bedside, he popped his stethoscope into his ears and began listening to the woman's heart, as he'd seen the interns and me do. When the nurse asked, "What do you think is wrong with her, doctor?" Irwin laughed and said, "I think she needs an operation." Then he wandered back into the corridor.

At about that time, one of the night nurses on the pediatric ward noticed that Irwin was not in his room and, after quickly searching the floor, called the hospital police. The security force, a little thin at that hour, spread out around the hospital. They finally located the lost patient banging on the candy vending machine outside the closed cafeteria. After the guard bought Irwin a Snickers bar, the patient gratefully returned to the pediatric ward. For the rest of his hospitalization, Irwin's room was locked from the outside when he went to bed at night.

I'd like to report that following that early morning consultation, the nurse on the internal medicine floor phoned the cardiac surgeon and Mrs. Jones underwent surgery that ultimately saved her life. I'd like to report that, but I can't. Not being on call the night of Irwin's elopement from the pediatric ward, I don't really know what happened to Mrs. Jones. Presumably, the nurse realized that the doctor who responded to her page was no doctor.

•

After awakening at home and dressing in his scrub suit, the on-call intern throws some essentials, such as a toothbrush, some toothpaste, and fresh scrubs, into an overnight bag and heads out the door. He will usually make it to the hospital by 7:00 A.M.

Reaching the hospital, the on-call intern's first stop is the coffee shop. There, by mutual agreement, he purchases breakfast for both himself and the intern who was on call the night before. Having successfully gathered breakfast, he then ascends to the ward on which he's working, his home away from home for the next thirty hours or so. After delivering breakfast to the intern who's finishing call and, in return, getting sign-out on his patients, the intern does prework rounds, making sure his patients have survived the night.

At 7:30, the day's flurry of rounds begin. Work rounds are followed by intake rounds, X-ray conference, and then attending rounds. Because of all of these rounds, the intern gets virtually no work done until noon.

While the morning and afternoon proceed, admissions begin to make their way up to the floor. The on-call intern is responsible for working up these patients, developing a plan of management, and, after reviewing it with the resident who's covering him, carrying out that plan. On days when there are few admissions, there's a reasonable amount of time available to get all the scut work that has accumulated done. But when the admissions begin to pile up (as they usually do), life can get pretty horrible.

It goes on like that through the night. Sometimes, there's no letup, and the house officer remains awake and working all night. On some nights, however, when admissions are few and the scut work is easy, the intern might manage to sneak off and get some sleep in the on-call room.

Nothing more than a glorified, semi-private flophouse, the on-call room is a disgusting place, an untidy, frequently smelly room that's packed with a bunk bed or two. Usually, the room's only other furnishing is a telephone, a necessity for answering middle-of-the-night pages. And, like a flophouse, the man or woman sleeping in the bed next to you (or on top of or below you) is often a stranger, someone you may have seen and even spoken with while at work, but about whom you know very little.

But getting to bed is more an exception than the rule. On most nights, there are so many admissions and so much work that needs to be done that there's barely enough time to make it to the bathroom. And after being pelted with a constant barrage of newly arriving admissions, by the time the rest of the ward team arrives to begin prework rounds the next morning, the intern has just about had it. With no sleep, no time to shower or even brush his teeth, all the intern wants to do is crawl off and die somewhere.

Unfortunately for the now post-call intern, dying is not yet possible at that hour. Before he can be relieved, the intern must sign out the patients to his resident and co-interns, go on work rounds with the team, and, because he's going to be called on to present new admissions, stay around at least through the conclusion of attending rounds. At that point, about noon on most post-call days, the intern is finally free to sign out his patients to the intern who's going to be on call that night and go home. Of course, if there's still some scut work that needs to be done, progress notes to write, or doctor's orders to renew, the post-call intern might decide to stay around a little longer so that he doesn't have to dump this extra heartache on his colleague. And so, the post-call intern winds up staying a few more hours.

Being post-call is an interesting experience—not a good

experience or a nice experience, but an interesting one. Spending a night working without any sleep strips away the subtle veneer of social skills that people normally take for granted. The post-call intern has trouble controlling his emotions—sometimes he'll become giddy, laughing and giggling at almost anything even slightly humorous; at other times, he'll become tearful, crying at the drop of a hat. Having lost his sense of tact, he'll tell you exactly what's really on his mind, never considering the consequences of those words. As a result, most fights between house officers and staff members occur on post-call days. Being post-call and having to function is an uncomfortable, uncontrollable feeling.

When he's finally had a chance to leave the hospital, the post-call intern wants to do nothing more than go home and get into bed. Unfortunately, there are forces that might prevent that from happening. He has to deal with those around him, the significant others and children who, having had their own lives put on hold for the last two days, want and deserve a piece of the house officer's time. In addition, there are obligations that must be fulfilled, errands that must be run, things that can only be accomplished during the day. Through all of this, through all these distractions, the intern's thoughts remain on reaching that elusive goal: sleep.

Unable to stay awake any longer, the post-call intern collapses by 7:30 in the evening. He sleeps through the next morning when, not yet refreshed but needing to get to work, his alarm clock goes off. During the second post-call day, the intern will go to the hospital in the morning and stay on the ward, finishing the work that got put off the day before, trying to prepare for the day to come. And then, if the intern is on call every third night, by the time the next day rolls around, it's time to begin the whole cycle again.

As a result of this schedule, interns are capable of having virtually no social lives. They're too tired to go to concerts or movies, they can't concentrate on reading newspapers or books, and, except for reruns of *The Odd Couple*, they don't watch much TV. If forced by family members or significant others, they'll occasionally consent to go to weddings and similar festive events, but they're almost always too tired and disconnected to ever have a good time. Even when they get together with friends and loved ones, there's virtually nothing they can discuss other than medicine. It makes for very boring conversation.

On a Sunday in March of my internship year, I was forced to attend the wedding of one of Beth's cousins, a woman I'd never met and whom Beth hadn't seen in almost ten years. I'd been on call the day before and had been up that whole night. The wedding was held in New York, and so, after being relieved, I drove to Logan Airport and caught a shuttle to LaGuardia.

The flight had been bumpy, and I'd been nauseous and couldn't fall asleep. By the time Beth and her father picked me up outside the terminal, I was pretty much a basket case. We drove directly to the catering hall. In the bathroom, I washed my face, shaved, and changed into the suit Beth had packed for me before she'd left Boston the day before. Fully dressed but feeling awful, I joined Beth and her family in the chapel and waited for the ceremony to begin.

Sitting in the pew, I tried desperately to stay awake while the rabbi droned on about these two people who were complete strangers to me. I did pretty well, considering; I only fell asleep twice during the ceremony. Beth wouldn't have awakened me either time, except she said my snoring was beginning to drown out the rabbi's words.

After the ceremony, Beth led me into the dining room and sat me on a chair between herself and her mother at our table. I drifted off into a dream state, staring at the fruit cup that had been placed on the table before me. I sat there, staring at that fruit cup, undisturbed, for a hell of a long time. Eventually, a waitress appeared, asked if I was done with my fruit, and, when I didn't answer, the thing disappeared. I was doing all right; I figured I could survive this as long as neither Beth nor her parents expected anything from me.

But then the band began to play a horah. The music was so loud, I could feel teeth vibrating. Upon hearing the rhythmic music, a lot of people got up and formed a circle in the center of the dance floor. The bandleader, not satisfied, yelled, "There are still people sitting. I want everybody up!"

This brought a few more people to their feet, but I didn't budge. "I said everybody!" the band leader repeated, pointing to our table. Embarrassed, Beth rose and pulled on my hand. Without putting up much of a fight (there wasn't much fight left in me), I got up and let her lead me to the circle.

I saw the man go down. He was old and heavy, and he probably shouldn't have been dancing so vigorously. I was on him almost before he hit the ground. It was all reflex; it couldn't have been anything else.

I checked for the pulse in his right carotid, but couldn't feel a thing. My father-in-law reached the man almost as soon as I did. As I went for the chest, he cleared the airway. I began external cardiac compressions, counting, "One one-thousand, two one-thousand . . ." out loud, as I'd learned in my basic life-support course. My father-in-law performed mouth-to-mouth resuscitation, blowing air into the man's mouth every time I reached five one-thousand.

I was aware that the band had stopped playing, that a crowd had formed around us. At some point, a man announced that he'd phoned the rescue squad. Beth helped slip my jacket off, and I was now pumping in shirtsleeves. But the only thing I was concentrating on was the man's condition. He looked fine, pink and alive, as long as I pushed down hard on his sternum. But whenever I stopped to feel for a pulse, there was nothing. For all intents and purposes, he was dead the moment he hit the ground.

It might have been different had the hall been equipped with rescue equipment. The man might have survived had we been able to start an IV and shoot some epinephrine into him. But no drugs were available. It was just my father-in-law and a very tired me breathing and pumping, breathing and pumping, over and over until relief arrived.

After a while, the rescue squad came in. Using a cardioverter, they tried to shock the man's heart, but it didn't work. Eventually, with my father-in-law still giving mouth-to-mouth and me still beating on the man's chest, the paramedics put the man on a stretcher and led us out of the hall. "You know he's dead," the head paramedic said after we'd passed through the hall's main entrance.

"I know," I replied. "He was out the minute he hit the ground."

"I didn't think it was a good idea to declare him in there," the head paramedic said. "What is that, a wedding?" I nodded my head. "This guy's a relative?"

My father-in-law said, "Yeah. He's the groom's uncle."

"It ain't such a good sign," the second paramedic said, "having your uncle die during your wedding party."

They'd finished putting the body in the back of the wagon by this point and then drove off. After washing up in the restroom, my father-in-law and I went back into the hall where, to our amazement, the party had resumed full tilt. Dinner was being served, but I wasn't hungry. I just stared at my plate of roast beef and little potatoes for what seemed like another hour. After a while, I asked Beth if it wasn't getting late. She said we could leave, and my father-in-law drove us back to the airport. We caught the shuttle back to Boston, and Beth drove our car back to Watertown. I was in bed by 9:30 P.M., and I slept soundly until the next morning when I had to get up and return to the reality of internship.

House officers frequently find that people who aren't in medicine don't, in fact can't, understand what's happening to them. There's no way to explain being up all night caring for sick and dying patients to someone who's never lived through that experience. Eventually, they wind up limiting their contacts to include only other house officers.

Scott Lindsay realized this very early in his internship. Here's a small portion of his diary entry of July 4, 1994, following his very first night on call in the NICU at West Bronx Hospital:

After finishing the night, I rounded with the people who were coming on for the day. Then I finished my notes and drove straight to my girlfriend Renee's apartment. I picked her up, and we drove out to my uncle and aunt's house in the Hamptons for their annual Fourth of July party. It was a nice party, but I was so tired and disoriented I couldn't really enjoy myself.

Of course, everyone asked me, "How was it? How was your

first night on call?" The last thing I wanted to do was recount everything that happened, being up twenty-nine, thirty, thirty-one straight hours (I can't really calculate it accurately at this moment), working with all those horrible premies in the NICU. So I just told everyone it was fine, everything was fine, and I didn't go into any detail.

I found that I couldn't really carry on a conversation with any-one. These were people I'd known my whole life, my parents, my aunts and uncles, my cousins, and I had the feeling that no one understood what had just happened to me. So I just kept to myself and, eventually, after lunch, I snuck into one of the bedrooms and just fell asleep.

That wasn't such a great thing to do; I mean, Renee didn't know most of these people, she was meeting a lot of them for the first time, and for me to disappear like that, leaving her without anyone she knew to talk to, it wasn't the most outgoing thing I've ever done. I think she understood. She knew how tired I was, and how irritable, but still, it wasn't a terrific thing to do.

Anyway, I was so tired that we didn't even stay for the fireworks, which is the high point of the whole day. We left at about seven o'clock and Renee drove us home. It's now 9:30, and I'm going to sleep. And this is only my first night on call. What am I going to be like six months from now? Oh man, I might as well just resign from the human race.

Part 3: Res-Speak: The Language of the House Officer

Between the publication in 1965 of *Intern*, by Dr. X, the first true account of the life and experiences of a house officer, and *The House of God* in 1978, a startling change in the language spo-ken by interns and residents occurred, a change that, unfortunately, reflected a greater depersonalization and loss of respect for patients than had ever before existed.

To some extent, a degree of depersonalization already existed by 1960. During his rotations on the surgery service, Dr. X again and again referred to patients on whom he'd operated in terms of the diseased organs that had been removed. Here's a brief excerpt from Dr. X's diary entry of Thursday, December 15:

> Today—Thursday—was fairly routine and not much excitement. Scrubbed with Emery on a gallbladder, the fastest damned gallbladder I've seen yet, forty-five minutes from start to finish. . . .
>
> Forgot to mention that . . . parotid tumor case Wednesday night . . .

But Dr. X, who refrained from using medical slang as much as possible, always showed respect for his patients, never belittling them because of their infirmities. In *The House of God*, this respect had largely vanished. Again and again, the hospital's staff, led by the hero of the story, the resident known as the Fat Man, belittle and disparage patients, referring to them not as diseased organs, but in far more insulting terms. Old people transferred to the House of God for acute medical attention from neighboring nursing homes are routinely referred to as GOMERs (an acronym for "Get Out of My Emergency Room"); old women whose mental capacity is at a slightly higher level than that of a GOMER are called LOLs in NAD (for "Little Old Ladies in No Acute Distress").

But *The House of God* did not create this language and these emotions; Samuel Shem reflected the attitude at hospitals around the country. There were slang terms that I heard used (and used myself) daily in the hospitals at which I trained that did not appear in Shem's book, terms such as GORK (an acronym used for patients whose mental status was damaged, standing for "God Only Really Knows"), horrenderoma (a patient with a horrible disease that had a terrible prognosis), fascinoma (a patient with an interesting disease or finding), and SHPOS (the worst of these slang words; reserved for abusive patients who are held in the most contempt, the term is an acronym for Sub-Human Piece of Shit).

These terms, this lack of respect for those who are their charges, has crept into the house officer's vocabulary for one reason: Interns and residents see patients as the enemy. It's as if a war is being waged in which the medical staff is on one side and hospitalized patients are on the other. As the house officer views it, the spoils of this war is sleep (no surprise there). The patient prevents the house officer from sleeping.

In addition to the disparaging terms interns use to refer to their patients, there's a medical shorthand spoken by house officers that is virtually incapable of being interpreted by members of the nonmedical community, a language house officers use to insulate themselves, to prevent their patients and families from understanding their words. They'll say a patient has a lethal condition rather than say the patient is dying; after death, they'll tell loved ones the patient has expired (leading the family to believe that everything would be okay again if they could only renew him).

The words we use—the insulting terms for referring to patients, the medicalese we employ to insulate us against patients, in fact, much of what composes the residency subculture discussed above—are nothing more than symptoms of an underlying disease. Most medical students come to medicine because they want to do something with their lives to help their fellow man. Humanism and idealism are good and important traits in young doctors, attributes we should recognize and build upon during their training. But instead of building on them, instead of fostering their growth, the process of turning a student into a doctor—the unmercifully long hours, the unforgiving hard work and desperate situations, the misery and depression and death—actually contributes to their destruction. We ultimately come to view the patients we once wanted to help as the enemy; we come to recognize their cries for help as attempts to prevent us from getting to sleep.

Unfortunately, things haven't changed in the years since *The House of God*. Here's part of a diary entry from Scott Lindsay, dated February 16, during his second and final rotation on the children's ward at Mt. Scopus:

Two of my patients are ultrachronic, unstable GORKs, both with uncontrolled seizure disorders, congenital malformations, and, to put the cherry on top of the sundae, with bad asthma and unstable airways. It's very rewarding caring for these kids. What a sense of satisfaction I get from treating them when they get sick and unstable! I spend hours and hours with them, and, eventually, I stabilize them enough so they can return to their original underlying state of GORKdom.

One of these kids, an eighteen-month-old with GM1 gangliosidosis [a rare inherited disease that causes progressive degeneration of the central nervous system; similar to the better-known Tay-Sachs disease, individuals with this condition usually die by the age of three], *is a real gem. She gets worse and worse every day. Now she responds to pain, but to almost nothing else. She just lies there all day having seizures and developing pneumonia, and there's absolutely nothing we can do. When she has a seizure, she has these apneic episodes where she stops breathing. Each time this happens, which is five or six times a day,* the parents come running, yelling at us to come quickly and do something, and by the time we get into the room, the episode is over and she's back to normal. Then the parents yell at us like it's our fault, like we're withholding some treatment from her that's causing all this to happen.

It's gotten to the point where I'm really having trouble dealing with these people. I know they're going through a lot and I understand it can't be easy watching your kid get worse and worse every day, but come on, it's not my fault! Last week, I had to restart her IV. I brought all the stuff into her room and the parents crowded around me and started cross-examining me: "Are you good at this? How many IVs have you put into patients?" I wanted to say to them, "What the hell difference does it make? She's so neurologically wasted, she barely moves when you stick her." But I didn't; I told them I'd started a lot of IVs. Then I managed to get it on the first stick.

5

NOVEMBER

The Fifth Rotation:
The Viral Syndrome

A few years ago, when a patient presented with symptoms and signs like lymphadenopathy [enlargement of the lymph nodes] *or hepatosplenomegaly* [enlargement of the liver and spleen], *we used to have a long differential diagnosis. We used to consider dozens of medical conditions that might be responsible for these symptoms and signs. Now in the Bronx, if a kid comes in with either of these conditions, he's got the viral syndrome until proven otherwise.*

Richard Andrews, M.D.
Director of the residency program in
pediatrics at Schweitzer

I remember the first time I drew blood from an actual patient. It was the summer of 1977, I was a third-year medical student, and I had just started my first clinical clerkships, a seven-week rotation in pediatrics. Matt Winston, the intern to whom I'd been assigned (and the man who told me never to get into a fight with a lab technician or an elevator operator), asked me to get some blood from a patient named Randy Rivers, a six-year-old boy who had glycogen storage disease, a rare inherited disorder that causes, among other problems, low blood sugar.

Having never drawn blood before, I was more than a little nervous. But Randy was a terrific kid, friendly and amazingly cooperative. Although he moaned and said, "Oh no, not another blood test," when I told him what I had to do, he put up almost no resistance. He held out his arm and turned his attention back to the TV program he'd been watching before I'd entered the room. After rolling up the sleeve of his pajamas, I wrapped a rubber tourniquet around the boy's upper arm and, as I looked at his elbow, I saw something pop up in Randy's antecubital fossa. It was a vein, a large one, and I was pretty sure I'd be able to get a butterfly needle into it. So after getting everything ready, I passed the needle through the boy's skin with shaking hands. Randy yelped a little, but then rapidly returned to his TV program. Hesitantly, I nudged the needle forward until blood appeared in the tubing. Quickly attaching a 5-cc syringe to the needle's hub, I pulled back on the syringe's plunger until blood filled the empty tube to the 3-cc line.

I had done it! For the first time, I'd successfully drawn blood from a patient. As I removed the needle from the boy's arm and squirted the blood into a red topped tube, my heart nearly danced.

Unfortunately, my joy lasted only a few seconds. As I was considering whether to have this needle and syringe bronzed and made into a wall plaque, I heard Randy say, "You did a good job, Dr. Bob, it didn't hurt much. But is my blood supposed to be dripping out like this?"

Looking down at Randy, I suddenly realized that in my jubilation, I had forgotten to untie the tourniquet from around the boy's arm. By that point, blood had leaked down Randy's arm, saturated his pajama top, and made a large stain on his bed-sheet and blanket.

I managed to quickly cover up my screwup. After yanking off the tourniquet and covering the wound with a gauze pad, I got Randy out of his pajamas and into another pair; I stripped the bed and remade it, using sheets and a blanket stolen from the ward's linen cart. Then I threw all of the evidence down the ward's laundry chute. By the time I returned to the nurses' station clutching the red-top tube of Randy's blood, I'd recovered enough to turn this misstep into a complete success. I received cheers from my intern and his colleagues.

Looking back on 1977, I realize how much simpler life was when I was a third-year medical student. All through my training, I was taught that invasive procedures, although potentially unsafe for the patient, were completely safe for the doctor performing them. Wearing gloves while drawing blood or starting an IV was unheard of. Sheets and pajamas soiled with blood and other bodily fluids caused no concern; they could be mixed in and treated no differently from any of the other dirty linens. And although needles and syringes did need to be disposed of with a certain degree of caution, no one's life flashed before his eyes if a needle happened to accidentally pierce the skin of his finger.

It was in 1981, in the second year of my residency, that life for doctors and patients radically changed. In that year, in a single issue of the *New England Journal of Medicine*, a series of articles heralded the appearance of what appeared to be a mysterious new disease. The condition, which was associated with a rare form of cancer called Kaposi's sarcoma and serious and unusual infections such as *Pneumocystis carynii* pneumonia, appeared to cause destruction of the immune system. Affecting previously healthy individuals, this disease, which was originally known as GRIDS (for "Gay Related Immune Deficiency Syndrome") but ultimately came to be called AIDS, led to a rapid, downhill course with quick and unexpected death. Looking back, I remember thinking how this disease, which acted like no other I'd ever heard of, could significantly alter the entire way medicine was practiced.

Today, no house officer would consider drawing blood or starting an IV without wearing at least one pair of gloves. No one would perform mouth-to-mouth resuscitation without first insuring that the patient's secretions could not be inhaled. In emergency and operating rooms, doctors have taken to wearing full battle dress—complete with heavy gowns, layers of thick gloves, rubber masks, eye protection, and boots—before coming in contact with any patient. And a simple accidental needle stick can cause a major life crisis, producing weeks of psychological torture as the young doctor waits for enough time to pass to see whether he's now HIV-positive.

But HIV has changed a lot more than just the way we approach patients. The virus that causes AIDS has brought about major revisions in the way medical care and basic science research is financed. It's altered the way new, untested drugs are licensed by the FDA and brought to market. And it's changed the role of pediatricians.

Since the time that the specialty emerged in the nineteenth century, one feature that attracted young doctors to pediatrics was the fact that children rarely die. Most children, even those who become critically sick, could, with time and the proper supportive care, completely recover. The emergence of AIDS in the 1980s changed all that: Suddenly, sick children would enter the hospital critically ill, be diagnosed with *Pneumocystis carynii* pneumonia (PCP for short), and either die of their infection or get better. But even those who recovered would, over the course of the next few years, become sick again and again. Eventually, they all died. The pediatrician, who for so many years had mostly good news to tell parents, was suddenly placed in a position where bad news was being given out on a regular basis.

AIDS and HIV have even changed the language of medicine. For fear that patients and their families will freak out if they know the diagnosis is being considered, in the emergency room and on the wards of the hospital, the disorder is referred to simply as "the viral illness."

By 1986, the time the house officers portrayed in *The Intern Blues* began their training, the viral illness had already significantly changed the way young doctors were trained. In my March entry from that book, I wrote:

> Amy, Mark, and Andy, as well as every other intern and resident in our program, have each been involved with at least one AIDS patient. Over the past couple of years, about one child with AIDS has died every month [on the wards of our hospitals]. Occasionally, the death seems almost like a blessing; these children are alone, with no loved ones; they are comatose, lingering on day after day in a vegetative state with no hope of survival. But most of the time, the death of a child, any child, is a tragic, deeply disturbing, and anxiety-provoking event for the house officers, nurses, and other staff members who care for the child and who stand by helplessly watching, unable to do anything to alter the course as the child grows sicker and weaker until he or she ultimately dies.
>
> But the inevitability of the death of the patient is only one factor that's changing the way house officers

approach their charges with AIDS. The second and perhaps dominant force is tied to our current knowledge of the way in which HIV is transmitted. House officers know very well that if they stick themselves with a needle that has been in the vein of an HIV-infected individual, they can become infected. And becoming infected is equivalent to a death sentence.

Has anything changed in our experience with AIDS since the time of *The Intern Blues*? The answer is both yes and no. As was the case with Amy Horowitz, Mark Greenberg, and Andy Baron, each of the young doctors I followed in 1994 and 1995 had encounters with patients with HIV early in their internship that played a role in shaping their year. In late August, during the second month of her rotation at Jonas Bronck, Denise Powers took care of an infant named Monica Smith, a four-month-old who entered the hospital with what was thought to be bronchiolitis. The infant was found to have pancytopenia (a deficiency of all blood cells, including red cells, white cells, and platelets). Over her first few days in the hospital, rather than improving, Monica grew sicker, her breathing becoming more labored. Finally, it was decided to perform a bronchoscopy, a procedure in which a tube is passed into the trachea so that samples of sputum can be obtained for examination. On August 29, the results of the sputum testing became available. Here's Denise's diary entry from the next day:

I'm so damned drained and tired. Yesterday was not one of my better days. I had to tell Monica Smith's parents that she has AIDS. We got confirmation yesterday that the specimen from her bronchoscopy was positive for PCP. She has PCP, that's why she was so sick when she came to the hospital and why she hasn't gotten bet-

ter. We also found out that she's HIV-positive, and since she's HIV-positive and has PCP, that means she has AIDS. What a terrible, terrible thing to have to tell a parent.

I haven't felt this bad since I had to tell my mom that her own mother had died. When we sat in the room and talked, I cried along with the mother, like Monica was my own child.

Let me back up. We actually found out about the diagnosis on Wednesday night. The parasitology lab called to say they'd found Pneumocystis in the samples sent from the bronchoscopy. I told our attending, who immediately called the immunology lab to see if the HIV testing had been completed. The technician in the lab told her over the phone, "Oh yeah, that test was positive." Just like that, completely matter-of-fact, without any emotion or anything: "Yeah, that baby's HIV-positive. Anything else I can help you with?"

So we knew Wednesday night, but we decided to wait until Thursday morning to tell the family. The attending said it was easier to do that kind of thing during the day, when the social worker and other support people are around.

So that's how my day started out today. We arranged a morning meeting. Unfortunately, only Monica's mother came. So when I first told Monica's mother, she was alone. There were no other family members there. It was just her and me talking and, oh man, was that painful. Very painful. And afterward, everybody told me, "Oh, you did a great job in there."

Great job! Yeah, a great job! Oh man, I hope I never have to tell anyone else anything like that again.

I think what got me the most was, had it been something like leukemia or some other form of cancer, I'd only be telling the mother about the child. That's not easy, either, but with HIV, it means that not only is Monica positive, but so is the mother. Monica's father might also be positive, or maybe Ms. Smith got the virus from her former husband who died a few years ago.

And the trail goes on and on. If it had been her former husband who transmitted the virus to her, then that means that maybe some of Ms. Smith's older children might be infected, too. And that guy had children with another woman, so they all might be infected also. It's like, you make a diagnosis in a baby and suddenly whole families are wiped out. There's no end in sight.

One of the main reasons I decided to go into pediatrics was because so few children ever die. Most of the time, we give our patients a little Proventil or a little touch of antibiotics, and they get better and go home.

I never thought it would be like this . . . [crying]

I never thought it could be like this.

I came home from work last night and took a hot bath and went to bed. I was too depressed to even eat. Oh God [crying], I never thought internship would be like this. I wish none of this were true. I told that woman how I wished it weren't true. I wished with all my heart. But what good did it do?

Please God, never make me have to do anything like this again.

And in Denise's entry from the next week.

Monica Smith finally went home late last week. She started to get better as soon as we began treating her for the PCP. Unfortunately, I think we lost her and her family, because her parents were supposed to bring her back to the ward on Friday for me to do a CBC [complete blood count]. I made all the arrangements, but neither she nor her parents ever showed up. When it was clear that they weren't coming, I called their house twice, but I got no answer. She also had an appointment at the immunology clinic today, and I don't know if she showed up for that, either. I'm just afraid that, because they're in denial, they're just going to ignore all the medical appointments we set up for them.

That's terrible. I know, and they know, that we can't cure Monica of AIDS or take away the HIV infection from her body, but the fact is, there's a lot we can do to keep her strong and healthy for a long time. If she's cared for properly, she could live ten, fifteen years, easy. I just hope the parents don't shorten what could be a reasonably good life span just because they're afraid and in denial, or because they just don't want to deal with any of this.

I have the feeling I'll never see them again. I feel bad about how this all went. This was the first time I ever had to tell a family that their child had HIV. It was the first and, as far as I'm concerned, I'm praying really hard that it's also the last.

Unfortunately, Denise's intuition about the Smith family turned out to be correct. To this day, she hasn't seen Monica or either of her parents again.

In early September, while working on the infants' unit at Mt. Scopus, Hal Burkins also had the unfortunate task of telling a family that their child had AIDS. Hal's experience with this sad event, as detailed in his diary entry from September 10, was remarkably similar to Denise's:

I don't think I'll ever have as sad a day as I had today. I've been taking care of a three-month-old baby who was transferred from the ICU, where she was being treated for PCP. They'd drawn a test for HIV, and after she was stabilized, they sent her down to the floor to finish her treatment. We'd been waiting for the results of the blood test and today they came in.

The baby's mother gave her consent to have the blood drawn, but she hadn't told the father about it. The father's beaten her in the past, and at the time of the baby's admission to the ICU, the mother had gotten an order of protection against him. Apparently, their relationship had been over for a long time: The father's been sleeping around and only checks in to brutalize her about the way she's taking care of his daughter. So she was frightened about telling him that the baby was being worked up for HIV. She didn't know what he would do to her.

Anyway, we were continuing the treatment that was started up in the ICU, all the time never mentioning anything about the testing to the father. All he knew was that the baby was being treated for pneumonia and that she seemed to be getting better.

Well, as I said, the test came back today and, of course, the baby's HIV-positive. So this morning, we had to tell the mother.

Lourdes, the social worker, Dr. Sherman, our attending, and I asked the mother to come into Lourdes's office so we could discuss the baby's care. The mother said, "Okay." She looked scared and asked me, "Is everything okay?" I said "Yes." I didn't really want to bring it up in the middle of the ward with all the other children and their parents around.

We walked down the hall, and I could see the mother twirling her hairband in her hand. She was very nervous. She knew it wasn't necessarily a lead-pipe cinch that the baby had HIV. They told her upstairs when they got her permission to do the testing that there were other possibilities, other immunologic problems like SCID [severe combined immune deficiency syndrome] and di George syndrome [in which, among other congenital anomalies, an immune deficiency occurs], but she also knew that those disorders were rare and unlikely and that the most likely explanation for her baby's having developed PCP was that the kid was HIV-positive.

We walked into the social service office and all sat down, and the attending started talking. "As you know, we've been worried about the baby. She has an unusual infection, one that usually occurs in people who have a problem with their immune system. One of the things that can cause an infection like this is AIDS. So as you know, we sent off a test for HIV. We got the results of the tests a little while ago. I'm sorry to have to tell you this, but the test came back positive."

The mother sort of nodded, and then she swooned. I thought for a second that she was going to pass out, but she didn't. Then she began to cry, and pretty soon, she was convulsing with tears. Lourdes put her arms around her and hugged her, and the mother pretty much collapsed into the social worker's arms. We all remained silent for a minute or two. It seemed like forever.

After a while, Dr. Sherman went on to explain that it was important that we continue aggressively treating the baby's infection and that we keep her as healthy as possible for as long as possible. The mother nodded her head a little, but she still wasn't able to say anything. She was still crying.

Then Dr. Sherman brought up the fact that the mother needed to be tested also. He encouraged her to go to the medical clinic and get it done as soon as possible. I knew she had a negative test during the early part of her pregnancy with this baby. Because the baby's positive, the mother must also be positive, so she must have become infected with the virus during the later stages of the pregnancy.

After a few minutes, while still crying, the mother told us how scared she was about telling the father. She told us again how he'd beaten her, and she was sure that when he found out, he would go crazy and kill her. Dr. Sherman told her that we would help tell the father. Lourdes said we could get the mother into a shelter if she was worried about her safety. She also pointed out that it was important for the father to be tested as well. The mother didn't say anything. She just sat there crying. It was very painful to watch.

About then, Dr. Sherman and I left. The mother stayed behind, still hanging on to and hugging Lourdes.

Then this afternoon, the father came to visit. Remember, at this point, he didn't even know that we'd sent off an HIV test on the baby. I called Dr. Sherman, he came back up to the ward, and he and I took the father into Lourdes's office.

This time, I did the talking. "When the baby came into the hospital, we found out that she had a serious form of pneumonia called PCP. It's unusual for healthy children to get this kind of pneumonia. Because of this, when the baby was in the ICU last week, they sent off a test for HIV. We got the result back today. Unfortunately, it showed that the baby is HIV-positive."

The father was absolutely floored. He was so shocked and devastated, you could not believe it. "How did the baby get it?" he finally asked.

Dr. Sherman told him that it must have been passed on to her from the mother. "She may have gotten it from somewhere else," he told the father, "but she also may have gotten it from you."

The father told us there was nothing wrong with him. "I feel fine. I'm in perfect health." We told him that that was part of the tragedy of this disease, that it struck people who are perfectly healthy and in the prime of life, and that usually they don't feel sick or act sick and they may infect other people before they even know they have it. The father told us he'd never been tested.

The man really looked shocked. He was staring off into space. We asked him if he'd had any other partners, and he denied it (which I think is not true). He seemed incredibly frightened and was trying to digest the information, thinking about how his whole life might have just been completely changed. He was sort of groping for answers and trying to figure out what his place was in all this. Obviously, the baby has HIV and the mother has HIV, and there's a very strong possibility that he has it, too. Thank God his reaction was, "I've got to get myself tested."

Pretty soon, the meeting wound down. He never cried, he kept up a very strong front. Later, when I was back on the ward, I saw him and the baby's mother go off for a walk together.

Afterward, she told me what she'd said to him. She told him that, knowing his temper, she was afraid he might flip out and really hurt her. His response was, "No, I wouldn't do anything like that. You and the baby are sick, and now I've got to be here for you." Thank goodness he turned out to be more supportive than any of us expected. We'll see what happens in the days to come, but right now it's turned out better than we all anticipated.

The mother and father are going to go and get themselves tested tomorrow. Unbelievable. The baby will survive this episode and has a chance to live for a reasonable amount of time. But we all know that she's ultimately going to die of this disease. And what makes it worse is that she's a beautiful little girl. I've never seen such long, beautiful eyelashes on a baby before. And she smiles at me and she's happy. It's very sad that she's going to die.

There are two other AIDS babies on the floor. One of them, Caroline Nieves, is actually approaching the end stages of her disease. Caroline's three years old and she's very sick and cachectic; she looks like death. Her mother's also very sick; she's also dying. Caroline's mother is very devoted to her. She's in her room with her whenever she feels strong enough. It's as if they're both going to die soon, but neither wants to go first. The mother is hanging on so she can be there for her daughter, and Caroline's hanging on because she doesn't want to leave the mother alone. It's as if on some level, they both understand this and it's keeping them both going.

This is an awful, awful disease. It's unbelievable that what's happening to Caroline and her mother is what's waiting down the road for this little baby with the long eyelashes and her mother. It's hard to believe: in one day, two and possibly three death sentences. What a job!

It turned out that Caroline Nieves's mother's desire to remain alive for her daughter was stronger than Caroline's need to not let her mother down. Coincidentally, in February, during her first night on call on Infants', Denise Powers presided over Caroline's death. From her diary entry of February 2:

This girl's death was horrible. It went on all afternoon. The patient, Caroline Nieves, who had end-stage AIDS, suddenly began hemorrhaging. She was bleeding from her mouth, her nose, her rectum, everywhere. We worked on her for three hours. We intubated her, started lines, gave her blood transfusions, but nothing helped. We finally declared her dead at 4:20 P.M.

This girl was my friend Michelle's patient [Michelle was one of Denise's co-interns on Infants' that month]. *I took the death worse than Michelle did, though. I have a lot of trouble dealing with children dying, and it doesn't seem to be getting any easier for me. Michelle took it pretty well. She told me that it usually takes her a few days for the news to settle in, and that she's sort of in a state of shock until that happens.*

The thing that makes it worse is that while you're trying to deal with the child's death yourself, you have to try to comfort the family. This baby's only family is her mother, who is also very, very sick with AIDS. The mother was extremely upset. Caroline's death wasn't unexpected, we all knew she was going to die, but it happened so suddenly that the mother wasn't ready for it. In watching her baby die, it was like this mother was looking into the future and watching her own death. Man, that was rough!

In October, during his rotation on the adolescent ward at Mt. Scopus, Hal Burkins cared for a patient mired in the end stages of AIDS. The interaction was to haunt him for weeks to come. The story begins with an entry from his diary dated October 10.

It's been a really terrifying week. Something happened this week that's really scared me to death, and I'm still not sure how I'm going to handle it.

I have this patient, Erica Jones, a fifteen-year-old with end-stage AIDS. This is a terrible story. Her mother died of AIDS when Erica was four. Since Erica was fine, everybody thought she was probably HIV-negative. Then, when she was seven, she developed acute kidney failure. Just like that, out of the clear blue, without any explanation. She was tested and found to be HIV-positive. She's been sick off and on since then, but it's pretty clear that over the last few months, she's really taken a turn for the worst.

The kid looks terrible, like warmed-over death; she's lost a lot of weight, she's not able to keep any food down, and she's on all sorts of medications. The immunology service decided that she needs to be put on TPN [total parenteral nutrition, which supplies all necessary nutrients intravenously] *and, of course, because she's been so sick for so long, she has no IV access left. So we decided it was necessary for her to go to the OR and have a Hickman* [an indwelling, surgically-placed IV line] *put in. The surgeons came and saw her and put her on the OR schedule, but they told us they'd only do it if we got her medical problems stabilized.*

Fine. So one day last week, I spent the entire day getting Erica ready for surgery. Everything was wrong with her: Her electrolytes were out of whack, she was anemic, and her clotting factors were all screwed up. I had to start a new IV, give her a transfusion of whole blood, play around with electrolyte replacement, trying to get everything just right, and, of course, at the end of all this, I had to take samples of blood and test that everything had normalized.

The big problem was, because she's been stuck so many times, she's become ultrabelligerent. Whenever I walked into her room to do anything, she'd get obnoxious and rude and yell at me to go away and leave her alone. So that morning, in a soft voice, I said back to her, "Please don't raise your voice. I've been very polite to you, all I ask is that you be polite back to me. You can be angry all you want and you can voice how you're feeling, but just don't raise your voice." She just rolled her eyes. Then I went ahead and did what I had to do.

Well, I put the new IV in, gave her the transfusion, gave her the electrolyte solution, and drew her blood for follow-up testing. Each time I went into the room, she kind of glared at me as if to say, "What the hell do you want now?" But my little talk with her apparently worked, because she didn't raise her voice to me again, and didn't say anything obnoxious or rude.

We got everything squared away, and the next day she went to the OR where the surgeons successfully put in her new Hickman. It's a relief to all of us, because now we don't have to keep sticking her to start new IVs or to get as many blood tests.

The day Erica went to the OR, my resident, Sam, took me aside and patted me on the back. He told me that the best thing that's happened all month was my arranging Erica's surgery. It was such a pain in the ass to everybody. He even told me that I deserve an extra day off for having done it. Of course, he wasn't in a position where he could give me an extra day off, but it was nice of him to tell me that. It really made me feel great.

Unfortunately, though, something really terrible happened the next day. You're not allowed to use a new Hickman for a few days until it heals properly, so I still had to stick her each time we needed a blood test. That morning, I went in to get a CBC [complete blood count] to make sure she wasn't bleeding internally as a result of the surgery. I got the blood, squirted it into a purple-top tube, and put the needle and tube on a table because she wanted me to pour her a glass of water. When I reached out to pick everything up, I somehow accidentally stabbed myself with the needle.

I stabbed myself in the left index finger with the fucking needle! I still can't believe that really happened. I was wearing the gloves I'd used when drawing the blood, so right away I prayed that the gloves had saved me, that the needle hadn't penetrated my skin. But it must have gone in pretty deep, because as soon as I tore off the glove I saw blood running out of the site. That's when I really started to panic. I thought, "Oh shit! I'm going to die. I'm already dead."

I was panicking. I didn't know what to do. I'd never stuck myself with a needle before. I've always taken precautions and been really, really careful about it. I ran out of Erica's room without saying anything to her and headed to the clean utility room, where I washed my hands with soap and started running tons of water over the wound. After a couple of minutes, one of the floor nurses came in to get something and asked what I was doing. When I told her I'd been stuck with a needle from Erica Jones, she said, "You'd better wash it with Clorox and go to employee health service." I did as she said and, within ten minutes, I was sitting in the health service's waiting room.

All sorts of things were going through my mind. I stabbed myself with the needle I'd used to draw blood from a patient with AIDS! I was clearly going to wind up infected. I was going to die an agonizing death. I'd never be able to finish my residency, never be able to practice medicine. And what was I going to do about Robin [Hal's wife]? What was I going to tell her? How was she going to deal with this? During that time I sat in that waiting room, I was really in a bad way.

After a while, I got to see the doctor. She calmed me down a little. She told me that studies have shown that the risk of contracting HIV from a single needle stick is much lower than was originally thought, less than 1 in 100. She drew my blood for an HIV test *(even though I had one a couple of months ago, just before starting internship), gave me a shot of immune globulin* [an attempt to kill off the virus before it has a chance to actually invade the cells of the immune system], *and told me I have to come back every few weeks to have the HIV test repeated. She said it'll be months before we can tell for sure whether I've contracted the virus or not.*

I came back down to the floor. By that point, attending rounds were almost over; I decided to skip them altogether, so I went to the nurses' station to try to get some of my work done. But I was still very upset and found that I couldn't concentrate. I mean, I know the health service doctor had been trying to reassure me, but I also knew that I wasn't going to be able to survive for weeks or months not knowing whether I was dying or not. I decided to go up and see Dr. Logan [Ned Logan, an infectious disease expert, is director of the inpatient service at Mt. Scopus]. *I know he's very smart, that he knows about this stuff, and I figured he might understand what I was going through.*

I found him in the hallway down by his office. I must have looked terrible, because he immediately asked me what was wrong. I told him I'd been stuck by a needle from Erica Jones, and he immediately pulled me into his office and closed the door. He reiterated what the health service doc said about the risk of contracting HIV from a needle stick being very low. He also said that he understood completely that the risk figures don't mean anything when it's you who have been stuck, and that this wasn't going to be easy for me. He told me that, for my peace of mind, it might be a good idea for me to take some AZT, because that had been shown to decrease the infection rate somewhat. Then he said it might also be a good idea for me to get some counseling, to go talk to someone who might be able to help me get through the next few months. I told him I'd take him up on the AZT, but that I'd have to think about the counseling a little. I have so little free time as it is, I don't see how I can fit a regular counseling session into my life at this point. He told me he'd always be around if I found that I needed to talk or needed some help.

Before leaving, we talked about the issue of possibly passing the virus on to Robin through sexual contact. He felt that the risk was very low, but just to be sure, he suggested we use condoms. I guess there's no other choice—except abstinence.

I don't know why, but I felt better after talking to Dr. Logan. I guess just knowing there's someone who seems to care is important. He was reassuring and he told me to come back if I needed him. I guess the only thing to do now is wait and see.

This isn't going to be easy.

It turned out that Hal's hard work getting Erica Jones ready for surgery had a very positive effect on the adolescent's life. Although her prognosis seemed dismal at the time, Hal spent the day correcting her electrolyte disturbance and transfusing her with blood. Although it seemed as if his work would prove futile and that the girl would die any day, Erica survived not only that month, but in fact for the rest of Hal's internship year. The Hickman line worked wonderfully, allowing Erica to receive enough total parenteral nutrition to put at least a little meat on her bones. In a better nutritional state, with more protein to help her fight off infection, Erica bounced back and improved. And in early January, with home nursing in place to help assure that her Hickman line remained intact and she received her ongoing TPN treatments, Erica left the hospital, returning to the apartment of her aunt, the only home she'd known since the death of her mother eleven years before.

Hal Burkins's problems also eventually sorted themselves out. Here's part of an entry from his diary dated November 20:

This morning, I finally got the report of the HIV test I took last week. I couldn't believe it actually took so long. I've been on pins and needles since they took the blood last Tuesday morning at employee health. Anyway, the important thing is that it was negative. What a relief!

This test being negative still doesn't mean a whole lot; I know I can convert to positive at any time between now and six months from now. But the longer you go without converting, the better the chances are that you haven't become infected. So having this test come back negative is really a good sign.

Of course, Robin's very relieved, too. We went out to dinner tonight to celebrate, and she told me how worried she's been for me since I stuck myself. She told me she didn't want to say anything, because she knew it would make me feel bad, but it's been on her mind constantly since I came home that day in October and told her what had happened.

I have to admit, having her say that made me feel better also. I've noticed there's been something different between us lately, some tension that had never been there before. I've thought up lots of reasons why that could be: I was using a condom, something I hadn't done before, and that certainly left something to be desired; I've become more and more exhausted and self-centered since starting my internship, and that certainly had to have had an effect; and, of course, I've been worried about whether I was infected and might potentially be passing the virus along to Robin. But having her finally admit how upset she was about all this made me realize that that had to play into the tension I've been feeling. We'll have to see what effect this negative test has in the next few weeks.

Hal had repeat HIV tests every six weeks for the rest of the year. Each test was negative. He had dodged the bullet.

•

As I've already mentioned, when it came to AIDS, the experiences of Denise and Hal were not that different from those of Amy, Mark, and Andy. What, if anything, was different between 1986 and 1994?

In thinking about it, I've come up with two important differences. The first can be considered the result of amazing progress in the area of drug research. Because of major and relatively rapid advancements in the care and management of patients, the diagnosis of AIDS in the mid-nineties means something very different from what it meant in the mid-eighties.

When Amy, Mark, and Andy were interns, the diagnosis of AIDS was a rapid death sentence with no chance of appeal. In most cases, the disease was rapidly lethal: Children like Monica Smith and Caroline Nieves would become sick and die within a matter of weeks or months. In the mid-nineties, because of advances in the treatment of the primary disease and its secondary consequences, patients survive and remain healthy for much longer periods of time. Children who are HIV-positive live at home, attend schools with other children, and wind up getting admitted to the hospital on far fewer occasions.

The second difference was one of evolution. Like me, Amy Horowitz, Andy Baron, and Mark Greenberg had known medicine before the dawn of the Age of AIDS. Amy, Mark, and Andy had entered medical school before the initial reports about AIDS appeared in the *New England Journal of Medicine*. Although they learned to take precautions in drawing blood and starting IVs in patients who had AIDS, they learned from individuals who themselves had never had to take such precautions. Amy, Andy, and Mark experienced medicine as the world changed; they straddled the pre- and post-AIDS eras.

Denise, Hal, and Scott learned and worked in only one of these worlds, the post-HIV one. As students, they learned medicine from interns and residents who'd never known anything different; as interns themselves, the three took patients with HIV as commonplace admission, taking their place alongside the asthmatics, the meningitics, and the other bread-and-butter admissions of general pediatrics.

What will the future bring? Judging from how far we've come in the last ten years, it's not illogical to think that by the time the interns of 2005 begin their training, a vaccine and/or cure for HIV will be available. Only time will tell, but it does seem possible that someday in the not-so-distant future, patients found to have HIV infections will be treated with a course of medication and released from the hospital cured of their disease. And, at that time, a needle stick such as the one Hal Burkins suffered will not evoke the panic it did in 1995.

6

DECEMBER

The Sixth Rotation:
Bell Commission?
What Bell Commission?

At the end of November of my internship year, I received the night-call schedule for the upcoming month in the mail. I was scheduled to work on the Children's Two, the pediatric infectious disease floor, and as I scanned the list of dates and names, I fully expected to see the name "Marion" typed after every third date.

That's how our residency program ran. In 1979, the majority of training programs in the Northeast featured an every-third-night-on-call internship year. But as I scanned the December schedule, I found what I believed to be a mistake. Near the bottom of the list, next to the dates "December 24" and "December 25," I found, typed in capital letters, the word "MARION."

Now, forget the fact that I was scheduled to work either Christmas Eve or Christmas Day. Working holidays was a fact of life to which most of us had grown accustomed. We understood that someone had to be in the hospital for patients on

Thanksgiving and Christmas and New Year's Day. But both Christmas Eve and Christmas Day? Two nights on call in a row? This couldn't possibly be correct. No one, not even Don Murphy, our ineffectual chief resident who was responsible for making up the schedule, could expect someone to take call on the ID floor, a place where almost anything could happen, two nights in a row. This had to be a mistake. It was too crazy to be anything else.

I immediately paged Don. When he called back, I said, "I just got the December schedule, and I think you made a mistake."

"Not you, too," Don said, annoyed that I was bothering him with something so frivolous. "Can't you guys just accept the schedule without arguing? This one wants this night off, that one wants that night off, what am I supposed to do? I can't make everyone happy. But do you guys care about how hard it is to make up a schedule like this? Of course not!"

"Don, I'm not arguing about being on call any one particular night," I replied, trying to cut him off. "I just think you made a little mistake. I'm scheduled to be on December 24 and 25."

"Yeah," he said when I stopped talking. "So?"

"You don't expect me to take call two nights in a row, do you?"

He sighed. "You didn't come to our last housestaff meeting, did you?"

I had to admit I hadn't. Since I'd made the decision to leave the program back in August, I no longer felt like a part of the housestaff, and I'd stopped attending all semirequired after-work functions. "If you'd been there," Don went on, "you'd have heard that we were trying something new this year. People are either going to work Christmas Eve and Christmas Day, New Year's Eve and New Year's Day, or two days in the middle. That way, everyone will be able to get a four-day mini-holiday.

Didn't you notice that you're not on call for about a week after your two nights in a row?"

I hadn't noticed, but hearing it now didn't exactly give me a warm glow. "You mean you expect me to take call on Children's Two for two straight nights?"

"Sure. You can do it."

"How about if I don't want to?"

"Well, to tell you the truth, Bob, I don't really give a flying fuck whether you want to or not. You didn't come to the meeting where you could have voiced your objections. I spent a lot of time coming up with this schedule, and I'm not going to change everything now, just because you're not happy with it. If you want to switch, go ahead and find someone who's willing to do it. But at this point, it's not my problem, it's yours, and I'm not going to help you solve it."

After thanking him for his help, I slammed down the phone. Not surprisingly, neither of the other two interns who were assigned to work on Children's Two with me that month had any desire to switch their schedules so they could work Christmas. With no recourse, I just went ahead and did it: I spent more than fifty-five hours straight working on Children's Two at the Boston Medical Center.

That year, December 24 fell on a Tuesday. As usual, I got to work at 7:00 A.M. that day and began the routine tasks house officers perform on regular weekday mornings. After prerounding on my patients (I had six at the start of the day), I went on work rounds with the rest of our ward team. At 10:00 A.M., Dr. Mann, our attending, came to make his rounds, which ran until about noon. After these formal activities ended, the two other interns finished their work as quickly as they could and signed out. It being Christmas Eve, they both had plans and wanted to get out of there as rapidly as was humanly possible.

So by 3:30 that afternoon, I was essentially alone. The other interns were gone, the medical students were on vacation, and the resident who was on call with me was also covering three other wards. He came to check in only twice that evening. That was it: just me, two not-very-happy nurses who would have much rather been home celebrating with their families, and about a dozen patients—children who, despite our best efforts to get them out of the hospital for the holiday, were just too sick to be discharged.

It would be difficult to find anything sadder than a pediatric ward on Christmas Eve. Christmas is a holiday for children, a holiday when families should be together. During the preceding days, the ward clerk and some kindly volunteers had spent hours covering every inch of the unit with tinsel and blinking lights. Near the nurses' station, there was a garishly decorated plastic tree and a large electric menorah. But in spite of all these carefully arranged, cheerful dressings, a feeling of helplessness hung over the place. Some of the children on the ward that night were infants, too young to realize how rotten a deal they'd received. But the others, sick though they were, knew that this was not how Christmas was supposed to be spent.

At least for most of the kids, Christmas Eve was improved by the fact that their families had come to spend the holiday, but like me, Andre Watson was alone that night. Andre, an eight-year-old from Detroit, had come to Boston the Friday before to visit his aunt and her family for the holidays. On Saturday, he developed a high fever. By Sunday morning, he'd become nearly comatose. Terrified that he was going to die, his aunt rushed him to our emergency room, where a spinal tap verified what the ER doc had suspected: The boy had bacterial meningitis, a serious, potentially deadly infection of the fluid that bathes the brain. An IV was started, massive doses of antibiotics were

pushed into his vein, and Andre was admitted for careful monitoring and completion of the course of antibiotics.

Although he'd been critically ill when he'd come up to our
floor, in the forty-eight hours that had passed, the boy's condition had significantly improved. On Monday, he awakened
from his stupor; on Monday night, his temperature returned to
normal for the first time in two days; by Tuesday afternoon,
although he was still pretty sick, he was alert enough to know
that it was Christmas Eve, that he was alone in a strange city,
and that he was terrified.

I understood that in order to survive two straight nights on
call, I was going to have to pace myself. I would need to get my
work done and get to sleep as early as possible. At around 6:00
P.M. that evening, I got an admission: a four-month-old girl with
a left-lower-lobe pneumonia. It took me about two hours to get
that baby—who was febrile and breathing rapidly, but otherwise not very sick—worked up and settled in. At around 8:00
P.M., I did evening rounds. My plan was to check all thirteen
patients on the floor and finish any scut that needed doing.
According to my plan, if there were no screwups, I'd make it
into the bed in the on-call room by 10:00 P.M. at the latest.

As the sickest patient on the floor, Andre had been placed in
the room at the end of the hall closest to the nurses' station.
Having started rounds at the other end of the ward, he was the
last patient I checked on that night. Because his condition was
contagious, Andre had been placed in isolation in a two-bedded
room. Upon entering, I found the boy lying in bed, crying to
himself. "What's wrong?" I asked as I checked his bedside clipboard.

At first, he didn't say anything; he just continued to cry. I
put down the clipboard and looked directly at him. "What's
wrong?" I asked. "Is anything bothering you?" He shook his

head. "Does it hurt where they stuck the needle in your back?" He shook his head again. "Does your head hurt?" Again that shake. "Is it because it's Christmas?

His crying increased. "I know, I know," I said, patting him on the shoulder. "It's Christmas Eve, you're sick, you're in the hospital, and you're all alone. Is that it?" He nodded his head.

"Is your aunt coming?" I asked. He shook his head and continued to cry. (I was to find out later that one of Andre's cousins was home in bed with the flu. Figuring that Andre would be well cared for by the hospital's staff, the aunt chose to remain home with her sick daughter, who would otherwise have had no one to care for her.)

I sighed. "Well, I know how you're feeling. At least a little. I'm all alone here, too. Do you think it would help if you could speak to your mother?" For the first time, the boy looked up at me. He nodded his head.

Although Andre's room had a phone, he couldn't make long-distance calls. And because he was still contagious enough to be confined to his room, getting him to the nurses' station, where long-distance service was available, was problematic. So, assuring him I'd be right back, I went out to the clerk's desk and, after finding his home phone number in the chart, called his mother in Detroit. I explained that although Andre was feeling better, he was terribly sad. I told her the only thing that would cheer him up was hearing her voice. She said she'd call right away.

By the time I got back into his room, Andre was cradling his phone's receiver to his ear. His tears were gone and he was smiling. I heard him tell his mother how much he missed her.

I don't know how long they talked. After seeing that my treatment had cured his problem, at least temporarily, I left the room, going back to get my work done. Half an hour later, having completed the scut that had been left over from earlier in the day, I stopped back in Andre's room on my way to the on-call room. The boy was sitting up in bed, watching some Christmas special on TV. "Do you feel better?" I asked. He nodded.

"Good," I said. "I'm going off to sleep now. If you need anything, just ask the nurse and she'll come get me. Okay?"

He shook his head.

"What's wrong?" I asked.

"My mother said . . . she said that maybe if I asked you, you might be able to stay in my room with me. In that bed." He pointed to the room's second bed.

"You want me to sleep in your room?" I asked. He nodded.

I smiled. "Okay. It is Christmas Eve, and we're both alone. Okay, I'll sleep in here. But we've got to go to bed right now. You've got to turn off the TV."

The television and room lights were off within seconds. In another couple of minutes, Andre's breathing had settled into a regular, undisturbed pattern. I nodded off sometime after that.

That night, mercifully, the nurses awakened me from my comatose state only once. At 4:00 A.M., just before her next dose of antibiotics was due, the beautiful IV I'd placed in the arm of the four-month-old with pneumonia infiltrated. I can't say restarting it was too much of an ordeal, though. By that point in the year, I'd become fairly proficient at putting in IVs, and despite the infant's screaming and squirming, I managed to get another line started on the very first try. After completing the job, I got back into the bed in Andre's room and slept undisturbed until 7:00 the next morning.

Andre was still sound asleep when I crept out of bed. I noticed his eyes opening as, picking up my clipboard, stethoscope, and beeper, I tried to sneak silently out of the room.

After taking a shower and changing into a fresh set of scrubs in the on-call room, I was back on the floor by 7:30. During the half hour I'd been gone, the place had come to life. The parents who'd come to spend the holiday with their children had broken out Christmas presents and torn wrapping paper, dolls, and battery-operated mechanical toys. For the first time, the place actually started to feel like it was a holiday.

My covering resident was sitting in the nurses' station, taking all this in. We began work rounds; together, we walked to the end of the hall, turned, and worked our way back. We stopped outside each room, checked the vital-sign sheet, briefly examined each child, then made plans for what needed to be done that day. On a sheet of paper attached to the top of my clipboard, I generated a fresh scut list that would have to be completed that morning.

By the time we made it to Andre's room, the boy was dressed and sitting up on his bed. The night before, I'd told him that in the morning his isolation would officially be lifted and he'd be allowed to leave his room and mingle with the other patients, and he was raring to go. When we gave him the news that he was cleared, he got up and, pushing the IV pole in front of him, headed straight for the ward's playroom.

For me, Christmas was busier than expected. I spent the whole day working, not even getting the chance to watch when Santa Claus (played by one of the critical care attendings) came ho-ho-hoing onto Children's Two to distribute presents. After finishing my scut and writing a brief progress note on each patient, the admissions started rolling in. During the day, I got four new patients, including one critically ill child, a four-year-old who, like Andre, had been diagnosed in the emergency room with bacterial meningitis. Getting these new patients settled, starting IVs and sending off blood work, writing orders and admission notes, took most of the day. By 8:00 P.M., as I sat in the nurses' station working on the last of the admission notes, I was fighting to keep my eyes open. Unfortunately, I lost the battle.

For the first time that year, I actually fell asleep sitting up while writing in a chart. My head came to rest on my folded hands and I just started snoring. When I awoke an hour later, I was surprised to find that a blanket had been thrown around my shoulders. Wiping the sleep from my eyes, I saw Andre standing about ten feet away. "Are you okay?" I asked.

"Yeah, I'm fine, Dr. Bob. Look what Santa brought me." He held up a huge magician's set.

"Andre the Magnificent," I said with a laugh.

"Are you okay, Dr. Bob? Don't you ever get to leave the hospital?"

I laughed. "I've got to stay all night again tonight. I'll be going home tomorrow. I guess I fell asleep."

"I know," Andre replied. "You were sitting there, snoring real loud! It sounded like someone was sawing wood. I put that blanket on you."

"That was a really nice thing to do, Andre. Thank you."

"I thought you were going to get cold."

After finishing the admission note on which I'd been working when I fell asleep, I sluggishly rose and trudged down the hall to once again make evening rounds before going off to sleep. Worried that I might fall asleep in the middle of the hall, Andre walked alongside carrying my clipboard, trying to help me as much as he could. When we were finished, I walked him back to his room. "I'm going to the on-call room to get some sleep now," I said.

"Can't you sleep in here again tonight?" he asked.

"I guess so," I said, falling back onto the room's spare bed. "You don't think my snoring will keep you up?"

"It didn't last night," Andre replied.

On Christmas night, I fell asleep before Andre. The nurses tortured me most of that night, awakening me six times. I finally got up for good at 6:30 on December 26. After taking another shower and changing into yet another set of clean scrubs, I sat in the nurses' station waiting for the rest of the team to arrive. I was never so happy to see any of my fellow interns!

During work rounds that morning, we redistributed the patients. I wound up being the primary doctor for four. I made sure that one of my patients was Andre Watson. Andre and I had become pals, we'd looked out for each other, we'd become a team, and I didn't want to break that team up.

That morning, I somehow managed to make it through both work rounds and attending rounds. I wrote notes on my patients and, by 2:00 P.M., was ready to sign out to the intern who was on call that night. Before leaving, I made sure to say good-bye to Andre, who was busy with the magic kit the critical-care Santa had given him. "You're finally going home?" he asked.

"Finally going home," I repeated. "I've been here for fifty-five hours straight. It's time to go get some quality sleep. I'll see you tomorrow."

Before I left, the boy told me to drive carefully.

Andre remained in the hospital for another week, finishing off his course of antibiotics. I discharged him to his mother, who'd flown out from Detroit to collect her son. Before they left, I told her to take good care of him, that he was a very special little boy. I sighed and smiled as I watched them walk out through the doors.

•

That December, when I bellyached to my father-in-law about having to be on call two nights in a row, he laughed and told me once again how spoiled I was. An orthopedic surgeon who'd trained during the mid-fifties, my father-in-law used to tell me stories about how he'd managed to survive being on call every other night. Throughout those years, he'd work thirty-six hours, come home and sack out for twelve hours, then return to the hospital for another thirty-six-hour shift.

I can't imagine how anyone could survive that intense grind. His schedule translated into a week consisting of roughly 125 hours of work. During off nights, there was barely enough time to do the laundry, let alone have anything resembling a social life.

Of course, the point was that, originally, house officers weren't supposed to have social lives. Interns and residents were supposed to be slaves to the hospital. The term "intern" was meant literally; house officers were supposed to live in dormitories within the hospital. As an intern, you were not permitted to be married or have children. Your meals were provided, your hospital whites were laundered for you, and for the privilege of working your butt off, you were paid next to nothing (my father-in-law got $50 per month; by the early 1960s, the period during which Dr. X, author of *Intern*, was training, the starting salary had been raised to a generous $75 per month).

The philosophy behind all this was that working hard for interminable hours was necessary for the training of good doctors. Medical educators strongly believed that living, breathing, eating, and drinking medicine was the only way to learn the art. Of course, those medical educators, who happened to also be hospital administrators, realized that there was another significant gain in practicing this philosophy: Having house officers work all those hours for so little pay allowed them to run hospitals for a fraction of what it might cost had they had to hire real doctors to do the work.

Where did this way of thinking come from? What kind of sadistic mind could have conceived of a system in which young professionals are forced to spend the best years of their lives slaving away in conditions that would not be tolerated by any other group? In order to answer this question, it's necessary to travel back to Baltimore in the late nineteenth century.

The concept of "internship" arose at Johns Hopkins Hospital in the 1890s. Prior to then, after completing medical school, young men (the profession in the United States was limited to men) who chose to pursue a career in medicine apprenticed themselves to an established physician or surgeon. Under the guidance of this individual, the young doctor was trained, eventually reaching a state of competence. At that point, he went off on his own, establishing his own practice and eventually taking in his own apprentices. The system worked as well as any other.

But in the 1890s, Johns Hopkins Hospital was facing a financial crisis. Unable to afford such luxuries as attendants to push gurneys, clean bedpans, and wash floors, the hospital's administrator and the dean of the medical school came up with what they believed to be a stroke of genius. Rather than having to apprentice themselves to some anonymous private practitioner, the hospital would allow all graduates of Hopkins to spend a year training at their famous hospital. And not only would the graduates be granted this privilege, they would be provided with clean uniforms, nutritious meals, and a warm place to sleep. And the cost of this extravagant training to the young graduate? It would be free of charge. What could be better?

By the mid–twentieth century, medical educators had actually begun to develop academic justifications for this insane system. No, they argued, the issue wasn't simply one of economics; to the young physician, interning was an educational necessity. Without a system that demanded such long hours, how could a young doctor come to appreciate the course of diseases such as diabetic ketoacidosis? Without witnessing firsthand the signs and symptoms with which the patient presents, how could he ever be able to identify the condition? Without following the response to insulin and intravenous fluids, how could he understand the physiology and pathophysiology of the diabetic state? In order to fully comprehend all aspects of this illness, it was necessary to closely observe the patient from start to finish of the course of the illness, a good thirty-six or forty-eight hours. These educators argued that without such lengthy exposure during one's training, it would be impossible to call oneself a competent physician.

By the time I began my training, this brilliant justification for what began first and foremost as a response to an economic crisis had become an ensconced component of medical training. Working more than 100 hours a week in installments of 36 hours in a row was a necessity. Forget the fact that after 18 hours the young physician's brain is so fatigued and exhausted that no rational thought can occur; ignore the fact that as the hours pass, the number of mistakes made by the overburdened young doctor increases exponentially. Internship is a rite of passage, a hazing ritual necessary for entrance into the fraternity of medicine.

So imbedded was the concept of interns working interminable hours that, back when I was a resident, it seemed impossible to change the system. When I wrote *The Intern Blues* back in 1985, I concluded that, although the system was horrible, we seemed to be stuck with it.

But my conclusion was incorrect. After *The Intern Blues* was published, a change did occur in residency training, at least in New York State. The change didn't come about as a result of medical educators suddenly realizing that they were performing a grave disservice to both young physicians and their patients. Rather, the change came from outside. Residency training as we know it was altered largely through the actions of a single man, an individual who came to believe that the system had caused the death of his teenage daughter.

The story of the death of Libby Zion at New York Hospital on March 5, 1984, is by now well known, chronicled in newspaper and magazine articles, in a highly publicized civil trial broadcast on Court TV, as well as detailed in books such as Natalie Robins's *The Girl Who Died Twice*. Then eighteen, Libby had been well until March 3, 1984, when she developed a slight fever and symptoms of an upper respiratory infection. Her condition worsened the following afternoon; her fever rose to 102° F, and that evening, while trying to sleep, she became restless, somewhat combative, and confused. Concerned, her parents called their private physician, who advised them to bring Libby to the emergency room at New York Hospital, where she could be evaluated by the staff doctor on call. Complying with their doctor's advice, the Zions brought Libby to the hospital; after midnight on March 5, she was examined by a second-year resident; eventually, a decision was made to admit her to one of the hospital's internal medicine floors for evaluation and treatment of fever of unknown origin.

What happened to Libby following her admission is still something of a mystery. The medical record shows that her doctor's orders, written at 3:00 A.M. on March 5 by Luise Weinstein,

M.D., the admitting intern, included prescriptions for Tylenol to be given every four hours for fever and a single dose of Demerol, a strong pain medication, to be given immediately. Libby's admission note reflects the thought on the part of the medical staff that the young woman's symptoms were at least partly hysterical in nature.

But Libby's course during the next few hours indicated that she was suffering from an organic, rather than a psychiatric, condition. The nurse's notes state: "Pt [Patient] with visible shaking, thrashing across bed, trying to climb across siderails . . ." The doctor's notes state that during this period, she exhibited bizarre, seizure-like behavior. To protect Libby from injuring herself, she was placed in four-point restraint, essentially lashing her down to the bed frame. When this failed to control her behavior, an attempt was made to have Dr. Weinstein come and reexamine her. Instead, at 4:30 A.M., Dr. Weinstein, overworked, overextended, and already exhausted from more than twenty-one consecutive hours of work, gave the nurses a verbal order to administer Haldol, a powerful sedative.

In the next hour, Libby's fever shot up to 103.5, a strong sign that she was suffering from a serious infection. Dr. Weinstein, contacted by phone at 6:30 A.M., ordered a cooling blanket and cold compresses.

Within ten minutes, Libby Zion's heart stopped beating. Despite attempts to resuscitate her, she was declared dead at 7:30 A.M.

At no time during her hospital course were antibiotics prescribed. At no time was a lumbar puncture performed to assess whether Libby was suffering from an infection of her spinal fluid. At no time during her life was the cause of her agitation adequately evaluated. The cause of Libby Zion's death was then, and is still today, uncertain.

•

There is nothing in life more tragic than the loss of a child. In response to this terrible tragedy, parents react in different ways. Some sink into depressions so deep they can no longer carry on with their normal lives. Some try to lose themselves in alcohol or other mind-numbing substances. Still others, vowing to make sure what happened to their child never happens again, take up arms, either literally or figuratively, against the instrument they believe was responsible for their child's death. Organizations such as Mothers Against Drunk Driving arose in just this way.

Sidney Zion's response to his daughter's death clearly fits into this latter category. Having been sent home after Libby had been admitted with reassurance that she was in good hands, Zion, an influential journalist, novelist, and attorney, was notified of his daughter's death by phone at about 7:45 A.M. on March 5. After sorting out the facts, Sidney Zion recognized that Libby received less than optimal care from Dr. Weinstein. He realized that Dr. Weinstein's problem was not that she was a bad person or an incompetent doctor, but rather that she'd been placed in an impossible situation by a system that was out of control. Clearly overwhelmed, Dr. Weinstein was an inexperienced doctor who had been given too much responsibility for way too long a period of time.

So Sidney Zion concluded that at least one of the factors that contributed to Libby's death was the institution of internship. He came to understand that young doctors should never be left alone to manage patients for thirty-six hours at a time. Further, he realized that such inexperienced people should not be allowed to make life-and-death decisions, unsupervised, at any time, regardless of how many hours of sleep they might have had the night before. Sidney Zion was convinced that had Luise Weinstein been better rested and better supervised, Libby would still be alive.

And Mr. Zion, in an attempt to prevent what happened to Libby from happening to any other parent's child, used his substantial influence to try to change this seemingly unchangeable system. Amazingly, he succeeded. Following a series of hearings and a grand jury report in late 1986, the New York State Department of Health organized an advisory panel to look into emergency services in the state. Headed by Bertrand Bell, M.D., a distinguished professor of medicine at the Albert Einstein College of Medicine, this group—known from the outset as the Bell Commission—after meeting for approximately six months, issued a series of nineteen recommendations to the New York Department of Health. Among the more important were:

1. Nonsurgical house officers should work for no more than eighty hours per week, the figure to be averaged over a four-week period.

2. House officers assigned to work on inpatient floors should spend no more than twenty-four hours during a single, uninterrupted shift.

3. Residents should have at least eight hours off between shifts, and at least one twenty-four-hour period off every seven days.

4. House officers assigned to an emergency room should work for no more than twelve hours in a row.

5. House officers should be supervised by attending physicians twenty-four hours per day.

The New York State legislature adopted the recommendations of the Bell Commission and on July 1, 1989, those recommendations, now known to all house officers either as "the Bell Commission regulations" or "the 405 regulations," went into effect in every residency program in New York State.

The Bell Commission regulations were met with vehement outrage by just about everyone involved. Virtually everyone in every part of the system hated them.

The earliest complaints were heard from hospital administrators, who cried about certain financial disaster. They argued that limiting the number of hours house officers could work to only eighty per week (imagine: *only* eighty per week; the equivalent of working a sixteen-hour day five days a week, the limited hours were fully twice the number worked by most other people) would immediately bankrupt hospitals. Not only would the hour limitation require that about 30 percent more house officers, physician's assistants, and nurse practitioners be hired to cover the shortfall, but hospitals would also now be required to pay attending physicians to staff all emergency rooms and wards twenty-four hours a day. There was no way, the administrators whined, that hospital budgets could absorb these costs without experiencing severe hardships.

Next, the directors of primary care residency programs, such as internal medicine, pediatrics, and family medicine, screamed that the regulations would both ruin their efforts to educate doctors and undermine the care of all patients. Post-call residents forced to leave the hospital twenty-four hours after entering would be deprived of the chance to attend conferences and lectures designed to educate them. There would be no way for these residents to make up the material they'd missed. In addition, the twenty-four-hour rule would prevent post-call residents from being able to sign out patients to the residents coming on duty the next morning. Educators argued that the new system would disrupt the flow of patient care, undoubtedly leading to a marked increase in oversight mistakes, and ultimately cause an overall worsening of medical care delivery in large teaching hospitals, exactly the opposite of the effect Sidney Zion had hoped to bring about.

Directors of surgery residency programs were perhaps the most outraged by the implementation of the Bell Commission's regulations. Having long claimed that the only way to train a student to become an effective surgeon is to have that student perform a large number of operations, they hollered that limiting the number of hours a house officer could work, which would limit the number of operations he could observe and perform during his training, was both ludicrous and counterproductive. Instead of limiting the number of hours surgical house officers worked, these program directors argued, the number of hours should actually be increased.

Finally, the senior medical students scheduled to graduate in June 1989, the people who would become the first group of interns to work under the influence of the Bell Commission's regulations, were scared to death. Afraid that their training would be undermined and jeopardized, frightened that they'd be forced, like the children of the Third Reich, to spy on their program directors and inform the authorities about irregularities in the schedules, uncertain as to what the regulations might mean to their future functioning as physicians, during the National Residency Match that occurred in the spring of that year, these interns-to-be chose to stay away from training programs in New York State in droves. As a result, 1989 was one of the worst years for intern recruitment in most programs throughout the state.

As I write this in 1996, more than seven years after the regulations were implemented, just the mention of Bertrand Bell's name continues to evoke strong negative responses from those who were involved in medical education in 1989. The work of his commission and its recommendations have become and continue to be the butt of many jokes. Older physicians blame the regulations for every problem that exists in medicine in New York today.

But in reality, by the time the interns who I followed in 1994 to 1995 began their training, the 405 regulations had already become something of a dinosaur, for the most part ignored by directors of training programs and trainees alike. During their assigned days on call, the interns I followed routinely broke the rules, working on the wards for thirty or more hours at a time, spending more than eighty hours per week in the hospital. A day in the life of an intern in December of 1994, five and a half years after the Bell Commission regulations went into effect, is represented in this excerpt from Scott Lindsay's diary, dated December 9, 1994:

Post call. I got only twenty minutes of sleep last night, but the most important thing is they were twenty quality minutes, between 5:30 and 6:00 this morning. I'm tired, and I guess you might say I'm also sort of cranky.

I got almost no sleep, and it wasn't even a particularly busy night. We got seven admissions, which is not a large number for Six-A [the pediatric ward at West Bronx Hospital]. *It wasn't that busy, but things just never seemed to stop moving.*

To tell you what kind of night it was, the most interesting conversation I had was with the father of one of my new patients, a little nine-day-old admitted with fever. He told me that he thought it was good luck to step in dog shit. He told me that one day he was walking down the sidewalk and accidentally stepped in a pile of fresh shit. He cursed to himself, tried to scrape it off, and then walked on. About a block farther down the street, he found a one hundred dollar bill lying on the ground. So now he thinks stepping in it is lucky.

I don't even want to explain how we wound up talking about stepping in dog shit, but it was that kind of a night. What can I tell you?

When this morning finally came, I found myself just stacked up with things that needed to be done after work rounds. I was pissed off because one of the things I had to do was go down to the X-ray file room and fish out a bunch of X rays that needed to be reviewed for not only my patients, but for some of the other interns' patients as well. I shouldn't have had to do that! One of the other interns should have gone down there and run that scut. But did anyone volunteer to go? Did any of them say, "No, Scott, you were on last night, you should just finish your work and get out of here?" Of course not!

When I got back from Xray, I still had a bunch of things to do. I had to change antibiotic orders on some of the patients I'd admitted, I had to write progress notes, I had to answer stupid questions asked by the nurses. At one point, I asked one of the other interns if she could help me so I could get out at a reasonable hour. She said she'd like to help, but she was too busy with her own work. Bitch!

So I sat there, chipping away at my mound of scut, sweating over doing all this worthless junk, having eaten nothing but a half a bagel in the last seventeen hours, having had very little sleep.

At 10:00, I went to X-ray conference and got into a fight with the radiologist about a patient who wasn't even on my team. Then when I got back to the ward, I found that my little nine-day-old, you know, the child of the dog-shit worshipper, had spiked another fever. I talked it over with my resident, and we decided to give the baby some Tylenol. I wrote the order, and a couple of minutes later, the nurse came up to me and said, "I can't give this baby Tylenol.

He's only nine days old. We don't give Tylenol to babies that young."

This, of course, led to a whole big fight. Just what I needed after I'd been up all night and just wanted to get my work done and sign out! I talked it over with my resident; she said to give the baby the Tylenol. The nurse spoke to her supervisor; she said not to give the Tylenol. So I asked the nursing supervisor how she could disagree with orders given by the doctors, and she said, "Do you know what's wrong with you? You don't respect the nurses' opinions enough." I said, "What are you talking about?" She responded, "These nurses have been working here for years and years. They have lots more experience with these babies than you do. And you don't believe them when they give you advice. You should respect these nurses. Someday, their experience could save your neck."

Eventually, we gave in and just decided not to give the Tylenol. I went to attending rounds, presented the patients I'd admitted from the night before, and finally got my work finished by about 4:00 P.M. I signed out and left the hospital at 4:30. A nice thirty-four-and-a-half-hour work shift. Terrific!

Bert Bell, eat your heart out!

And Scott's experience is in no way atypical. The diaries of all three interns have repeated references to thirty-or-more-hour days. Here's one excerpt from Denise Powers's diary, dated November 26, 1996, in the midst of a rotation on the general pediatric ward at West Bronx Hospital:

Oh my God, when is this cycle going to be over? I was post-call yesterday, and I didn't get to leave the hospital until 7:40 last night. Thirty-seven hours in the hospital; now that's what I call a bad day!

It was horrible. Thursday was Thanksgiving; I expected it to be quiet and peaceful, but instead I got about 100 admissions. They must have put a sign up in the ER waiting rooms around the Bronx saying: "Attention all doctors: Dr. Denise Powers is on call tonight on Six-A at West Bronx Hospital. Wouldn't it be interesting to see how many admissions she could do in one night before flipping out?" That's what it seemed like, anyway. . . .

I spent the whole day and night running around, admitting patients, writing orders, running scut. At about 5:30 yesterday morning, I finally couldn't take it anymore. Of course, I still had tons of work to do, but I didn't give a damn. At West Bronx, the work is never done; the place is a never-ending trail of red tape and paperwork. By definition, the scut can never get finished. If you think you've finished all the paperwork, you're either simple-minded or you've misplaced a couple of vitally important documents that need to be filled out immediately in black ink.

Anyway, at about 5:30, I told my resident I had to go lay down for a while. I went into the lounge, pulled up a sheet, and was immediately comatose. I slept until 6:30, when the resident from the other team came in to get sign-out.

And, of course, that wasn't the end of it. That's when the work day really began. We did work rounds, went to X-ray conference, had attending rounds. Then one of my patients had an anaphylactic reaction [a severe allergic reaction during which the patient's oral structures swell, there is respiratory distress, and the patient can actually die], *so the resident and I had to get him stabilized again. I followed this by trying to finish some of the scut I put off when I went to sleep that morning, and before I knew it, it was 6:00 P.M. and I still was nowhere near ready to sign out.*

Somehow, I managed to make it out of the hospital and get home. I was so tired, I was actually afraid to drive. So I walked around the corner, got myself something to eat, and breathed in some of the cold night air. By the time I got back to my car, I felt awake enough to drive. I made it home safely and promptly passed out.

What a night!

But perhaps the most blatant example of disregard for the Bell Commission regulations that occurred during that year happened in September 1994. It involved Scott Lindsay, this time during his first rotation on the infants' unit at Mt. Scopus. The story is detailed in his diary entry of September 21:

I'm once again post-call. It wasn't a bad night, but I had a really big problem this morning. It involved one of our patients, an infant with a hemangioma [a tangle of blood vessels which can reach extremely large size; hemangiomas are dangerous, because they can grow through and block critical structures such as the trachea, causing respiratory distress] *that keeps expanding and has essentially taken over her trachea. She has loud stridor* [a loud noise on inspiration] *and is having more and more trouble breathing. She's being transferred to Memorial-Sloan Kettering* [a hospital in Manhattan] *this afternoon for treatment with interferon, which apparently has been successful in shrinking these things in lab animals. It's experimental and only available at a few hospitals around the country.*

Anyway, because they were afraid something might happen to the baby during her trip into Manhattan, the chief residents decided that a doctor should go on the transport, just in case. So Dr. Miller, who's my attending, asked during attending rounds, "Okay, who lives in Manhattan?" I said, "Oh, I do, but I was on call last night, and I have my car here." He said, "Well, would you mind leaving your car here today, taking the ambulance into the city with the baby, and then taking the subway to work tomor-row?"

Mind you, I'm post-call, and Mike Miller is one of the directors of our residency program. And he's asking me to go on a transport after I've been post-call, which is a direct violation of the 405 regu-lations. And it's not even like this baby is my patient. She belongs to one of the other interns on my team.

This really put me in a bind. I didn't want to go on the trans-port. I had no desire to do it. I wanted to tell Dr. Miller how totally inappropriate I thought this was, what a difficult position he was putting me in. But this guy is really important to my training; he's my ultimate supervisor. And to have him ask me to do this, I felt really uncomfortable saying no.

As it turned out, I was upset for nothing. I didn't have to go on the transport. Andrea, the intern who's actually responsible for the patient, told Dr. Miller that she was really interested in the treat-ment and wanted to go watch it. So in the end, it turned out okay for me. But this total disregard for the Bell Commission regula-tions by one of the people who is responsible for instituting those regulations shows what contempt there is for those rules in our training program. What nerve to even ask! What contempt and nerve!

After witnessing the effects of the Bell Commission regula-tions for seven years, I have to agree with Scott's assessment. The regulations have not worked. They have not significantly improved the work lives of house officers, and by causing a breakdown of continuity and an obvious disintegration in the management of patients admitted to teaching hospitals, they have clearly worsened patient care. The system of incessant sign-ing in and signing out caused by the mandated restriction of hours has created a perpetual and dangerous game of telephone, in which information about the patient's lab tests, medications, and clinical status is frequently altered or lost. It is inevitable that patients will often fall through the system's cracks, winding up staying in the hospital for extra days because someone forgot to schedule a test, make an appointment, or order home-care equipment well enough in advance. And unable to identify a primary care provider from all the house officers rotating on and off the service, the patients often feel disenfranchised, as if they have no one to turn to, ask questions of, feel a bond with. Clearly, implementation of the regulations has brought about a deterioration in patient care provided at large teaching hospitals.

I'm sorry to have to admit this. From the very beginning, I was an advocate of the work done by Dr. Bell's commission. Back then, reform of the rules governing the archaic system of training imposed on young doctors was a necessity; unfortunately, today it continues to be one. Having caused more problems than they attempted to solve, the Bell Commission regulations simply don't work.

It is time to reopen the issue. The commissioner of the Department of Health in New York State must recognize that the regulations in their current form have failed and convene a panel of experts to reexplore how reform can best be accomplished. Clearly, artificially limiting the number of hours house officers are permitted to work is not sufficient to improve either the delivery of medical care to state's hospitalized patients or the lifestyles of interns and residents. Suggestions for new changes are included in the epilogue of this book.

7

J A N U A R Y

The Seventh Rotation: Doctor, Heal Thyself!

It's almost inevitable that during the course of a year, a normal human being will become sick at least once. Whether it's a head cold, the flu, or an intestinal virus, these illnesses are usually little more than an inconvenient pain in the neck for a young, healthy person. Producing no lasting harm, they wind up causing you to spend a few days in bed, drinking plenty of liquids and taking aspirin or Tylenol (at least this is the advice given in TV commercials; none of this is actually taught in medical school). In a few days, the infection runs its course, you begin to feel better, and life returns to normal.

But for sick house officers, this is rarely the way an illness plays itself out. Although they understand that working while they're ill is not a good idea, interns and residents hate to call in sick. They understand that there are patients who need to be cared for, scut that needs to be done, nurses to fight with, and attending physicians to get chewed out by. If they're not present, their colleagues are going to have to provide that care, do that scut, fight those fights, and suffer the psychologically damaging effects of that chewing out. As a result, in an attempt to spare their fellow house officers, unless they're actually dying (and in some cases, even then), interns come to work sick, spewing secretions containing infectious viral particles on their friends, patients, and everyone else with whom they come into contact.

Why would anyone, especially a doctor who presumably understands the consequences of these actions, react in this way? What would cause a reasonably sane, responsible person with a fever of, say, 103° F to leave a warm bed in order to come to work in the hostile environment of an inner-city emergency room? The answer is guilt: House officers are trained to feel guilty if they have to stay home from work. Because of the difficulty inherent in finding someone to cover for absent interns, this insane reaction is burned into them early in their training by the chief residents—the people in charge, the very people on whom the intern must depend for support. If an absence occurs among the troops, it is the job of the chief resident to find someone to fill in; since this is a nearly impossible task, it's clearly in the chief resident's best interest to make the absent house officer feel as guilty as possible.

This feeling of guilt associated with getting sick is nearly universal. It has changed little since the days when Dr. X did his training back in the early 1960s. Here's a short excerpt from his diary entry of February 15 from the book *Intern*:

> The weekend is pretty fuzzy, don't remember very much about it except that last Friday I got a wretched cold, runny eyes, runny nose and a nice irritative bronchitis, coughed and coughed and coughed in the operating room until Archie [one of the attending surgeons on Dr.

X's service] turned me out of there, told me to go cough on something else besides his surgery. Saturday morning I felt like the wrath of God, just ached all over. I thought about trying to con Alec or Luke [two co-interns] into trading weekends with me, but then decided to try the All-Purpose Cure first, went up to Second [one of the wards on which Dr. X worked] and begged a couple of APC's [aspirin, phenacetin, and caffeine tablets] and 10 milligrams of Dexedrine [aka speed!] and took them and presently began to feel at least alive. The nurse offered to give me a slug of penicillin, but I talked her out of some tetracycline instead, being a coward about needles, and by Sunday morning the thing seemed to be squaring away. I just didn't do anything I didn't have to do, and the weekend was relatively quiet, compared with the last couple.

Coughing on the sterile field in the operating room! Self-treatment with speed and antibiotics for what almost certainly was a viral illness (viruses don't respond to antibiotics)! Remaining in the hospital where he could infect staff and patients alike, rather than having someone else cover! What kind of medicine is this?

Unfortunately, I have to admit that my attitude toward illness was no better than Dr. X's. During my internship, I got sick only once. It was during January, in the heart of flu season. I was working in the outpatient department that month, and on January 18, when I showed up to start my shift in the emergency room, the waiting area was already packed with febrile kids who, like me, were stuffed up and sneezing and just basically feeling horrible.

By that afternoon, I'd developed a bad case of the flu—my

head was stuffed, I had a fever, and it felt as if my arms and legs each weighed a ton. What I needed to do that night was crawl into bed and quietly die, but I knew that wasn't going to happen. There was no one available to cover for me. So instead of doing what I knew was the right thing, I went to work.

I reported to the ER that afternoon and, very slowly, began to make my way through the pile of charts. As usual, I was working alone; in those days, pediatric interns assigned to the ER at Boston Medical Center were the lone representatives of the department within about a half-mile radius. There was no one with whom I could discuss my findings, no one I could ask for help. And I really needed help that night; I was so sick that my judgment was shot. So, terrified that I was going to make a mistake, I began to make my way through the charts, praying that there were no really sick children lurking in there among all these kids with the flu.

At about 6:30, I was examining a patient when the triage nurse paged me to the waiting room stat. Fearing that one of the waiting patients had suffered a cardiac arrest, I rushed out, ready (or at least as ready as I could have been at that moment) to begin resuscitation. Finding the room calm, I saw the nurse pointing to the waiting area's TV, which was tuned to the local news on channel 5. There on the screen, Mike Flannagan, a pediatric attending at the Medical Center and medical editor of *Channel 5 News*, was interviewing Dr. Neal Morgan, our director of infectious diseases. Getting closer to the TV, I realized they were standing in one of the patient rooms on Children's Two, our infectious disease ward, discussing the epidemic of Kawasaki disease, a mysterious and potentially deadly disorder that had recently hit the Boston area. "It starts out looking like a common strep throat," Dr. Morgan was saying. "The children have high fever that lasts for at least five days. They develop sore throats with redness of the mucous membranes. Their lymph nodes become swollen, they have skin rashes, and their hands and feet swell. Eventually, the skin around the fingernails begins to peel."

"Are there any long-term dangers associated with Kawasaki disease?" Mike Flannagan asked.

"Oh yes," Dr. Morgan replied. "A small but significant percentage of children affected with this disease go on to develop coronary artery aneurysms, swellings of the arteries that carry blood to the muscle of the heart. The swelling can cause weakness in the walls of these blood vessels and problems that may lead to heart attacks or even sudden death."

"And so it would be important for parents to have a doctor carefully check a child having any of the symptoms of Kawasaki disease?" Mike asked.

"Very important," Dr. Morgan answered. And then, full face toward the camera, he said, "If your child has any symptoms of Kawasaki disease, you should contact your doctor immediately or come to the emergency room at the Boston Medical Center." As my mouth dropped open, in large, easy-to-read white numerals, the ER's telephone number flashed across the screen.

This was all I needed. I was feeling lousy and already overwhelmed, and our senior expert in infectious diseases goes on TV and tells all the parents of Boston that if their kid has a fever, sore throat, or swollen glands, they'd better get over to my emergency room immediately or the kid might suddenly die. Every kid in Boston had fever, sore throat, and swollen glands that night, but they sure as hell didn't all have Kawasaki disease; they had the damned flu!

The phones started ringing almost immediately; the lines were blinking like the lights on a Christmas tree. My progress through the growing pile of charts was stopped as I tried to handle all those calls. Most of them were legitimate: I was able to dismiss some of them as nothing more than a mild case of the flu, but many I just couldn't decide about over the phone and had to advise the parent to bring the kid in as soon as possible. But some of the calls were ridiculous, providing evidence that Boston had at least as many loonies as any other city. One woman called to tell me that eighteen years before, her son had had the exact symptoms Dr. Morgan had described on the news. Instead of Kawasaki disease, though, she said the doctors who'd cared for him at the internationally famous Boston Children's Hospital (our crosstown rivals) had diagnosed the condition as leukemia. Although he'd received chemotherapy for five years and had long ago been considered cured, the mother wanted me to now make a retrospective diagnosis of Kawasaki disease so that the young man could be cleared of the "stigma" of cancer he had carried all these years. Another woman called and said that although her six-month-old daughter had neither a fever nor a rash, she seemed to be drooling a lot. The woman wanted to make sure that drooling wasn't a symptom of Kawasaki disease that Dr. Morgan had neglected to mention on the news broadcast. "No," I told her, "it sounds like your daughter's teething."

"Yeah, that's what I thought," she replied. "I just wanted to check."

On and on it went into the night, the calls continuing to come and all the children with the flu whose parents didn't want them to suddenly die of a heart attack continuing to register at the front desk. And even though I was popping Tylenol and guzzling liquid and ounces of decongestant, as the night wore on, I felt sicker and sicker. I doubted that I'd ever make it through to the morning. "Please God," I prayed at one point, "make all this go away."

At around 11:30, I took a call from a man who'd been watching the late news, on which Mike Flannagan's interview with Dr. Morgan had been replayed. He told me that his two-year-old son had a fever, swollen glands, and was complaining that he had a "boo-boo" in his throat. After listening to the story, and feeling as if I couldn't rule out the diagnosis of Kawasaki disease over the phone, I advised him to bring the boy in. "How do I get to your hospital, doctor?" the man asked.

And all at once, the answer to my prayers came to me. Without hesitation, I said, "Do you know where Longwood Avenue is?"

"Sure," the man replied.

"Great. The address is 300 Longwood Avenue. It's called 'Children's Hospital.' Just go in the ER entrance."

"Thanks a lot, doc," the man replied gratefully. "We'll be right over."

The solution seemed brilliant. Why should I, in my weakened state, be killing myself? From that point on, I just sent anyone who asked for directions over to the Boston Children's Hospital.

And it worked. Although the calls continued for a while longer, the siege of registering patients stopped abruptly at about 1:00 A.M. By 3:30, exhausted and ready to die, I reached the bottom of the pile of charts: I had seen them all! Retiring to the on-call room a happy man, I immediately fell into a coma. I slept until 8:00 A.M., when, having been awakened by my relief, I called Don Murphy, our less-than-sympathetic chief resident, and told him I was going home. I slept all that day and night and by the next morning, I was feeling well enough to at least return to work.

•

I got off pretty easy during my internship. I wound up missing only that one day of work as the result of illness, and although I was married and Beth became sick a few times, I never had to ask permission to stay home and take care of her during that year. The same wasn't true for Amy Horowitz, one of the interns whose experiences were documented in *The Intern Blues*. Amy, who started the year with a two-month-old baby and ended the year in the mid-trimester of her second pregnancy, not only had to worry about her own internship-acquired illnesses, but those of her daughter, Sarah, and the symptoms associated with early pregnancy as well. When you consider all that she had to be concerned about, her surviving the year relatively intact was, at least to me, an amazing feat.

For example, on a Monday afternoon in March, Sarah, who was then nine months old, started getting sick. That night, the child woke up screaming and was found to have a temperature of 103.4°. Amy checked her, discovered she had a runny nose, conjunctivitis [inflammation of the sclerae, or white part of the eyes; also called "pinkeye"], and a cough. She gave her some Tylenol, rocked her for a while, and eventually Sarah fell back to sleep. From Amy Horowitz's diary entry of February 2:

> *She woke up again at 2:00 A.M. She was screaming and her temperature was back up. I gave her more Tylenol and tried to calm her down, but this time she just wouldn't stop crying. I was sure she had meningitis and told Larry [Amy's husband] to get dressed, because we had to take her to the emergency room, but just as he finished getting his clothes on, she quieted down and fell back to sleep. I guess the Tylenol had kicked in. Anyway, she slept the rest of the night, but I didn't; I stayed awake in her room, watching her constantly. I was sure something terrible was going to happen.*

On Tuesday morning, she woke up in a much better mood and her fever was gone. . . . When Marie [Sarah's baby-sitter] *came, I told her about what had happened and made sure she knew how much Tylenol to give if the fever came back. I was going to be in clinic that morning and was scheduled to be in the ER that afternoon and night, so I left Marie a list of phone numbers and the schedule of where I'd be, in case she needed me.*

I should have called in sick, but I went to clinic anyway. Marie called at about 10:30 to tell me that Sarah's fever was back and that she now had a rash all over. I told her I'd be home in a few minutes and I rushed through the rest of my clinic patients, just so I could finish. . . . I ran home to find Sarah's fever was back up to 103. She was miserable; she was coughing and sneezing and covered with snot, and she had a whopping conjunctivitis. And she had this raised red rash on her face and chest. I wasn't sure what it was, so I called Alan Cozza [Sarah's pediatrician and, in those days, the director of pediatrics at Jonas Bronck Hospital]. *He told me to bring her right over.*

Well, to make a long story shorter, Alan took one look at her and said, "My God, she's got the measles!" I'd never seen anyone with the measles before; kids don't get them anymore because we immunize against them. Alan brought some of the other interns who were on the floor to see Sarah, just so they'd know what measles looked like. I have no idea where she got it. She's a baby, she doesn't go outside, she doesn't hang around with other children, except sometimes when Marie takes her down to the lobby, but that's rare. But anyway, she had the measles. Alan told me to take her home and give her Tylenol and fluids and make her as comfortable as possible and that it would pass in a few days.

By that point it was nearly one o'clock. I was supposed to be in the ER starting at one, and since I was on call that night, I knew I'd be staying until maybe three or four in the morning. So I decided to stop in and talk to the chief residents. I figured, hearing that Sarah was so sick, they'd naturally say, "Well, why don't you just stay home with your daughter tonight?" Yeah, right!

What they said was that two residents who were supposed to be on call that night had already called in sick, they'd had to pull one person from the emergency room to cover the floor, and, although they sympathized with me, they just couldn't let me have the night off. If I didn't show up, there'd only be two house officers to staff the entire emergency room, and they just couldn't allow that to happen. They told me I should try to switch with someone who was scheduled to be on the next day, if I could find someone who would be willing to switch, but there was just no way they could give me the night off.

How nice of them! After all the abuse I've taken. . . . After everything I've done for them! Whenever they've asked me to do anything, I've always done it without a whimper! I've filled in for people, I've covered wards I'd never even worked on before because somebody was out, and I never complained. I've repeatedly put my job ahead of my family, and this is the thanks I get! The one time my daughter is sick, the one night I need to take off in order to be with her. Of course, no one would lift a finger to help me. I asked everybody if they'd switch, if they'd cover for me this one night, and they all had some excuse. I should have just gone home. I should have taken Marie and Sarah home and stayed there, and when they called to find out where I was and why I wasn't in the emergency room, I would have said . . . I don't know exactly what I would have said. But of course, I didn't do that. What I did was, I brought Sarah and Marie home and went back to the hospital. . . .

Well, it was a horrible night and I finally managed to get out of the emergency room at about four in the morning. Larry was still wide awake; he hadn't gotten any sleep, having been up with Sarah all night. Her fever was still over 102, and she was extremely irritable. She'd sleep for maybe a half hour and then wake up howling. She's never even had an ear infection before this. It's so strange seeing her this sick. . . .

I was all set to call in sick on Wednesday, but Larry had already made arrangements to take the day off, and he told me that I should go in. So I went to work, and when Alan Cozza called me in the morning to find out how Sarah was doing, I gave him a piece of my mind! I told him about how the chiefs had made me work the night before. He seemed shocked. He said he'd go have a talk with them, but a lot of good that does me! I'm really so angry. I'll tell you, this episode has really taught me a lesson. Let them ask me to do anything, let anybody ask me to cover or to switch; my answer is going to be "NO!" I don't care what it is or who it is, I'm not doing anything for anybody ever again! I've had it with these people! I've got to look out for my own interests, because no one else will!

This diary entry was made about a week before Amy went on the second vacation of her internship year. When she returned from that vacation in Florida, she was pregnant. I don't know for sure if Amy's pregnancy was the result of her anger with the chief residents, if spite might have played a role in her decision to become pregnant with a second child so soon after her first, but the fact is, by early May, she was suffering enough from the consequences of morning sickness that she had to announce to those chiefs that she was expecting and would need some time off.

The system's response to the needs of pregnant residents is actually one of the areas that has undergone significant positive reform over the past four decades. In the first half of this century, when relatively few women were admitted to medical schools, residency training programs didn't have to worry about developing specific policies about maternity leave. For most of this period, even the "problem" of giving male residents a few days off for paternity leave wasn't an issue, as, prior to about 1950, house officers, male or female, were officially forbidden to marry or have children during their years of training (unofficially, sex was undoubtedly discouraged as well). But since the 1960s, as women entered medicine in more significant numbers, those in charge of residency programs were forced to reexamine this situation. Changes have occurred, but they haven't come about easily.

Back when I was a resident in the early 1980s, pregnant women were clearly discriminated against. In December of my senior residency year, Delia Lederman, one of that year's interns who was then in the second trimester of her first pregnancy, developed deep vein thrombosis, a not uncommon complication of pregnancy. The formation of a blood clot in a vein in the leg, deep vein thrombosis is dangerous, because at any moment, a portion of that clot can break off, travel to the lung, and block blood flow to a significant portion of that organ, a condition known as a pulmonary embolus. As a result of this complication, deep vein thrombosis is a disorder that must be taken very seriously and aggressively treated.

In an attempt to prevent the clot from growing and spreading, in addition to bed rest, anticoagulants (sometimes called "blood-thinning agents") are administered to patients. Unfortunately, because it is teratogenic (that is, can cause birth defects) warfarin (also known as Coumadin), the most convenient and widely used anticoagulant, is contraindicated during pregnancy. As a result, another drug, heparin, is administered to pregnant women with this condition. But although heparin is safe to use during pregnancy, unlike warfarin, which can be taken by mouth, heparin must be administered intravenously two or three times a day throughout the remainder of the pregnancy.

So in December, Delia Lederman, who had completed nearly six months of her internship, was placed on bed rest at home; an IV was inserted into her arm, and for the remaining four months of her pregnancy, she administered injections of heparin into that IV every eight hours. Following the birth of her healthy son and, simultaneously, her recovery from deep vein thrombosis, Delia took an additional six weeks off, calling it maternity leave.

To say that Delia's pregnancy-induced absence engendered anger and rage from her fellow interns would be something of an understatement. Since our residency program had no system in place to deal with this situation, there was no one to cover for Delia during the months she spent away from the hospital, no official replacement to take her nights on call or to pick up her patient care responsibilities. Instead, her responsibilities fell on the interns and residents who were assigned to the wards on which Delia had originally been assigned. So instead of being on call every third night, those interns were forced to take call every other night; instead of covering one-third of the twenty-five or so patients on a ward, those interns had to cover one-half of them. Naturally, Delia's co-interns were not happy with this situation. And they didn't blame the chief residents or the directors of the residency program for their discomfort; they blamed Delia and her pregnancy.

Having experienced this situation, I have to admit that, although the situation was bad prior to the birth of the baby, things got a whole lot worse after Delia delivered and, rather than rushing back to work, opted to take those extra few weeks off to be with her newborn. Most of the other interns understood bed rest and IVs; they knew that working with deep vein thrombosis would actually put Delia's life in jeopardy. But they didn't understand why they had to continue working their asses off while Delia took what they viewed as a vacation?

When Delia Lederman finally returned from maternity leave, her life was misery. She was made to feel like an outcast by the rest of her fellow house officers. No one would talk to her, no one would help her out when she was having difficulty with a patient. It was horrible to watch.

The fallout from Delia's absence was felt throughout our training program. The consequences of this pregnancy taught the program's directors that a formal, written plan needed to be developed and adopted. It taught other women in the program that becoming pregnant could stigmatize them (one of the other interns, a close friend of mine who became pregnant soon after Delia Lederman delivered, actually managed to keep her pregnancy secret from the chief residents and most of the other residents until nearly the end of the second trimester; no one said a word as her wardrobe transformed or her body shape changed, and in spite of some horrible morning sickness, she never missed a day of work). And it taught Delia Lederman that no one really cared about her. Like Amy Horowitz, possibly to spite the chief residents who not only failed to help her out when she needed it but added to the spirit of animosity that ran rampant through the residency program, Delia became pregnant again during the latter half of her second year of training. Again, four months into this pregnancy, she developed deep vein thrombosis. And again, much to the disgust of the rest of the housestaff, she spent a nearly six-month period out of the hospital.

•

By early May 1986, when Amy Horowitz announced to the chief residents that she was pregnant, the situation had changed significantly for the better. But Amy's announcement wasn't exactly met with loving kindness and open arms. Here's part of her diary entry for that momentous day, May 11, 1986:

Jon and Arlene [two of the chief residents] *were sitting at their desks, and I walked in and said, "Hi. Guess what! I'm three months pregnant. I'm due next November, and I need to arrange maternity leave." Just like that. You should have seen the looks on their faces. I thought Arlene was going to fall out of her chair. Of course, whether I'm pregnant or not doesn't make any difference to them; they're not going to be here after June 1, so it isn't going to be their problem. It'll be the new chiefs' problem. But they certainly were stunned just the same. It took them about five minutes to recover enough to congratulate me. In some ways, it was worth suffering through these weeks of nausea and exhaustion just to see the looks on their faces!*

Anyway, what they've done in the past is that a three-month period of maternity leave has been created by taking the one month of vacation and the one month of elective without night call we're entitled to and adding another month of elective with night call. I told the chiefs that that was what I wanted to arrange, but they immediately started giving me a hard time. They said that as far as they knew, all I could get was my one month of vacation. They were unwilling to give me the other two months; they told me three months off would cause enormous problems in the schedule, and they just couldn't afford to do that. I've found out since then that three other women are pregnant and expecting at about the same time I am, and if they give us all two or three months off, it just might destroy the schedule.

Well, I don't care if my having a baby does destroy their precious schedule! I'm finished worrying about everyone else! What it comes down to is they're trying to discriminate against me, and I'm not going to just sit back and stand for it this time! I'm tired of being pushed around and doing things just because the chief residents or the attendings or someone else tells me that that's the way it has to be! So I made a call to the Committee of Interns and Residents [the house officers' union]. *I got one of the vice presidents on the phone and asked him exactly what the policy was for maternity leave. He told me that I'm entitled to six weeks of leave above and beyond any vacation or elective time I might have coming. That means that what I'm really entitled to is six weeks of maternity leave, four weeks of vacation, four weeks of elective without night call, and another four weeks of elective with night call. That's a total of four and a half months. And you can be sure I'm going to take advantage of every minute of it! If they hadn't tried to screw me . . . I would have settled for three or maybe even two months. Now I'm going to take four and a half months, and if they don't want to give it to me, I'm just going to file a grievance with the union!*

Following her discussion with the chief residents, Amy had a meeting with Mike Miller, the director of the residency program. Mike apologized for the way the chief residents had initially handled the situation and explained that, of course, she would be guaranteed two months of maternity leave and that the rotation to which she'd be assigned in the month prior to her due date and the month following her return would be low-stress ones. This placated Amy; in the end, she never filed a grievance and actually had a nice maternity experience.

Our residency program's current maternity leave policy has been working well. The policy has been carefully crafted to avoid problems such as those that occurred when Delia Lederman had her babies. As was the case with Amy Horowitz, pregnant women are allowed two months of time away from the hospital following the birth of their babies; they are usually assigned to "light" clinical services (i.e., those, such as electives, that do not carry with them patient care responsibilities on a ward) during the months prior to and following their maternity furlough. Coverage is provided, so that no other house officer is forced to suffer as the result of the birth of a baby. There's even been some joy built into the experience for a house officer: Following the birth of the infant, the family is sent a gift from the department, a specially designed baby blanket. These changes haven't solved all the problems that occur during pregnancy: Female residents are still overworked, exposed to potentially teratogenic infectious agents such as cytomegalovirus and teratogenic drugs such as Ribovarin [an antiviral medication used principally against an agent called respiratory syncytial virus; Ribovarin can cause birth defects when used around pregnant women, so care must be taken when administered], and are usually malnourished. Still, having this policy in place has at least relieved some of the psychological burden that these women were previously forced to bear.

None of the interns I followed in 1994 and 1995 became directly involved in a pregnancy during that year, but they did suffer from an assortment of illnesses. They each became sick, and each missed at least a few days of work as a result of that illness. The worst illness occurred to Hal Burkins. Near the end of his rotation in the outpatient department in January, Hal developed a case of the flu far worse than the one from which

I'd suffered. In my case, although I missed part of one day, I was left with no significant residual problems; I got sick, rested at home for a day, recovered, and came back to work, none the worse for wear. Hal Burkins's case of the flu was the proverbial straw that nearly broke the camel's back. His illness led directly to a depression that almost caused Hal to suffer a psychotic break in early February.

8

F E B R U A R Y

The Eighth Rotation:
Intern Suicide Season

That T. S. Eliot might have been a hell of a poet, but he sure as hell never did an internship. April is the cruelest month? It's not even close. If he'd done a year with us, he'd have realized that April's a piece of cake compared to February.
        Jesse Sherman, M.D., former chairman of pediatrics,
                    Albert Schweitzer School of Medicine
            (during a spontaneous discussion of T. S. Eliot's
            "The Wasteland" during attending round, 1981)

Jesse Sherman, a remarkable pediatrician and one of my mentors, was nearly eighty years old when he made the statement quoted above. Despite his advanced age, Dr. Sherman's judgment was as sharp as it had been a half century before. He knew that February is hell for house officers spending a year working in a hospital in the northeast United States. Ironically, although it's officially the shortest month of the year, to interns and residents, it always feels like the longest.

There are many reasons why February is so horrible. First, there's the weather. It's the dead of winter, it's freezing cold, and in New York, a generous layer of hard-packed, dirty snow covers the sidewalks and streets. The combination of the cold weather and this covering of frozen crud that makes walking even short distances dangerous keeps people perpetually indoors, the start of a recipe for the development of cabin fever.

Second, the periods of daylight are very short. Because they have to arrive at the hospital by 7:00 A.M. and often wind up running scut until well after 6:00 P.M., for most house officers, February is spent in a world of darkness. Incredibly, during winter, interns get to see the sun only on the weekend day when they're not expected to be at work.

Although the cold weather and lack of sunshine are elements with which all Northeasterners must cope, there are other, special concerns that exclusively affect house officers. By February, interns have been slaving away for seven months. As previously mentioned, the "thrill" of being an intern has long worn off and been replaced by the dull, chronic exhaustion that comes from working between 80 and 100 hours a week (or more, in some cases) and being on call and awake in the hospital every third or fourth night. By February, lacking enthusiasm and chronically overtired, house officers have used up all their stored reserves and are running on empty.

Making matters worse, the end of all this is nowhere in sight. In February, the conclusion of the academic year is still more than four months off. When you're tired, cold, out of shape, unable to exercise or even get out of your apartment to take a walk, four months can seem like an eternity.

Add to this the fact that the nature of the work they're doing is not exactly causing them to turn cartwheels. House officers work with sick patients. And although it's true that most of the patients an intern is responsible for get well and leave the hospital, some don't get better—they grow sicker and get transferred to an intensive care unit; some ultimately die. And when interns lie in bed at night after a long day at work, it's not the patients who've improved on whom their minds fix; it's the patients who've died.

By February, most house officers tell you that they feel alone, that because of what they've seen and what they've gone through, they're unable to communicate with their friends, their families, sometimes even with their significant others. As a result, whatever social lives they might have had prior to beginning their training have by February completely dissipated.

Finally, add to this the fact that February tends to be one of the busiest months in the hospital, and that, because it's flu season, a lot of interns and residents themselves become ill, and it's not hard to understand why more psychotic breaks and suicides that affect interns and residents occur during this month than during any other.

Given that February is so gloomy, how is it that anyone survives? Why do some interns make it through without difficulty while others fall apart? The answer is that, by this point, most house officers have developed successful coping mechanisms to help them make it through the bad times.

There are probably as many coping mechanisms as there are house officers. Many of these defenses are clearly destructive. Some house officers turn to drugs (which is not surprising, since, as doctors, they have easier access to controlled substances than do other people) and alcohol to numb the pain and blot out memories of the past and prospects for the future. Others become belligerent, blaming the directors of the program or their fellow house officers or even their loved ones, who are just trying to help. Yelling and screaming about how someone else is ruining your life can do wonders to improve your mood.

But there are many coping mechanisms that are positive and not at all destructive. For instance, some house officers rely on a healthy sense of gallows humor to help them make it through some of the absurd situations that occur during particularly bad days and nights. Some rely on inner strength, brought about by religious convictions, to help guide them. These interns and residents usually survive February intact.

Unfortunately, some house officers never develop coping mechanisms that can carry them through the most difficult of times. These residents are the ones who are the most worrisome; during February, these are the people who tend to crumble.

Each of the three interns whose diaries composed the book *The Intern Blues* had well-developed mechanisms for coping with stress. Amy Horowitz used two: As her greatest help, she relied on the support of her husband and infant daughter, but when times got the roughest, like when her daughter developed measles and she had to work, she chose to take out her hostility on those around her, especially the chief residents, whom she blamed for everything that was wrong in her life. Andy Baron used intellectualization as a defense mechanism, much the way I did during my own internship. For instance, he'd make lists of things that were right and wrong with his life and use those lists to justify in his own mind that he'd made the right decision by coming to the Bronx to do his internship. He concluded that his unhappiness wasn't due to any difficulty within himself, but with the system.

It was clearly his sense of humor that helped Mark Greenberg get through his first year of training. As is detailed in his diary entries, he was able to make jokes even during some of his most horrible moments. But even Mark's ironic humor nearly failed him in February when he worked in the NICU at

Jonas Bronck Hospital. He started the month in his usual, cheerful manner. Here's the start of his first diary entry of that rotation, dated January 27, 1986:

Today was my first day in the nursery. What fun I had! I love staying until 10:30 P.M., running around like a chicken with its head cut off, having no idea in the world what the hell I'm doing. It was a million laughs! I can't wait to go back tomorrow!

By the end of the month, Mark's tone had changed substantially. Here's his last NICU entry, dated February 25, 1986:

I haven't recorded anything in a couple of weeks. I look upon these tape recordings as a kind of funny running monologue, but I haven't felt very funny over the past weeks. Working in this unit has been terrible, just terrible, much worse than I ever imagined. We've had a lot of deaths and, even worse, we've had a lot of survivors, babies who should never have been allowed to live. I don't want to think back on what's happened, I just want to look ahead.

Every month so far there have been a lot of bad memories, but there have also been good ones, funny stories I'll carry with me probably for the rest of my life. This month, there have only been bad memories and worse memories . . . I've been finding that I just can't defend myself against them. It's been just brutal.

I don't want to make this sound too sappy, but I knew I was in trouble when I cried in the hospital last week.

Last Thursday I'd been up all night with this PFC'er [persistence of the fetal circulation, a serious complication in sick newborns, especially premies or infants who have aspirated meconium, which causes it to become impossible to deliver oxygen into the bloodstream of the baby] *who had done really poorly, and when he finally died, I just couldn't take it anymore.*

I went into the bathroom, locked the door, and just cried my eyes out. I'm really starting to fall apart. That was the first time I'd cried all year. . . .

Maybe sometime in the future I'll be able to come back to this and fill in some of the blank spaces I've left, but I can't do it right now. I need a nice vacation. I think I'll take my vacation in the West Bronx emergency room over the next four weeks [Mark's March rotation was in the outpatient department at West Bronx Hospital].

I'm going to sleep. Maybe when I wake up, things'll start being funny again.

They did. By the time Mark made his next diary entry, he was back to cracking jokes, laughing at a system that made little sense. But Mark clearly was humbled by February; his month in the NICU scared him, it knocked some of his self-confidence out of him, and as far as I could see, significantly altered his outlook on life and his work.

Two of the three interns I followed during 1994 and 1995 developed good protective defense mechanisms. Like Mark Greenberg, Scott Lindsay used his tremendous sense of humor to help get him through. Time after time, he made jokes out of some of the ridiculously absurd situations in which he found himself. For instance, in August, while working on the ward at West Bronx Hospital, he was asked to take care of a rather delicate problem:

The day after I was on call last time was doctor order renewal day. I had a lot of patients, so it took me until after 7:00 P.M. to get my work done. I finally finished, I was exhausted and was about to leave, when one of the nurses came up to me and said that the girl-friend of a seventeen-year-old patient with sickle-cell disease who's not even one of my patients (he belongs to an intern on the ward's other team) was visiting him and they were, to use the nurse's words, "making babies." The nurse walked in, caught them, and told them to cease and desist immediately. They just slammed the door in her face. Now she was coming to me, telling me it was my job to get them to stop.

Right! It's my job to get the patients to stop screwing each other. What do I care whether they're making babies or not? As long as they're not pulling out each other's IVs. That's all I care about. But having sex? Who cares? It may even be therapeutic; it'd probably take this patient's mind off his painful sickle-cell crisis.

Well, anyway, I saw that this nurse wasn't going to leave me alone until I did something. So I went to the microphone of the intercom system which is located in the nurses' station and announced into that patient's room, "Attention, attention. Please be advised that according to the West Bronx Hospital's Patients' Bill of Rights, which is posted for your reading pleasure on the wall by the elevator, baby-making is strictly forbidden within the confines of the patient rooms on the pediatric unit. If patients are caught making babies, they will be banned from the hospital indefinitely. To repeat: Baby-making is prohibited. Thank you for your attention."

I switched off the intercom, gave them about two minutes to get themselves together, and then I went into the room. The guy's girl-friend was now completely dressed. I told them I had been sent to check on them, because I'd heard there had been some hanky-panky. The kid said, "Who told you?" I said, "One of the nurses." He said, "Why? Isn't she getting any?" I said, "Julio, the point is, *you're in the hospital. No one's supposed to be getting any." Having made my point, I got him to promise not to make any babies while he was a patient on our ward. When I got back to the nurses' station, all the nurses were huddled together. The one who'd sent me in said, "So? Are you going to throw him out of the hospital?"*

I said, "I can't throw him out of the hospital. There was nothing going on."

"But I caught them," she said.

"Well, they've stopped. I'll tell you what. I'll write an order in the order book: 'Patient not allowed to have sex.' That's the best I can do."

And that's what I did. I wrote the order. Now if one of the nurses catches him, they can take it up with their supervisor. Amazing.

In addition to her sense of humor, the thing that saved Denise Powers during her most difficult times was the amazing support she received from her mother and her large number of friends. Through most of her diary, Denise told stories about dozens of people, none of whom I knew; I didn't even understand how most of them fit into Denise's past. Some were family members, some were friends from her old neighborhood in Brooklyn, while others had become close to her during medical school. Nearly all of these people had a tremendous understanding of what Denise was going through. They had the ability to comfort her when times became bad. It's safe to say that, at least a few times during her internship year, the love and friendship Denise received from these many people saved her hide.

But Hal Burkins had little of this. In reviewing his diary entries, there are clear indications from early on that he was headed for problems. In early November, Hal fixed upon a proposed minor change in the residency training program that had recently been announced and viewed this as a major threat to his education. From his diary entry of November 5:

I'm really upset. I just left Jonas Bronck after being on call. I didn't have a very good night. Nothing really bad happened, but I just feel frustrated. I'm not very happy with the direction this residency program is taking. We had our first intern retreat yesterday. Overall, it was good, a day off from work at a nice restaurant where we could get together and bond with each other while having a chance to bitch and moan about anything at all that was bothering us. We got a chance to talk about problems we thought existed in the program, things that we wanted to see changed. At the end of the day, the director of the program came and listened to our issues.

Serendipitously, it was revealed to us that starting in January, they're going to eliminate subspecialty clinics from the ambulatory care rotation. When that happens, all of our time during that rotation will be spent in the emergency room and in our continuity clinic [that is, the general pediatric clinic].

I think this is terrible. They're doing it strictly for economic reasons. New York State is trying to encourage all of us to go into primary care. They're funding nurse practitioners to take up the slack and do the scut work in the subspecialty clinics so that we can spend more time learning to be primary care pediatricians.

Well, that's fine. Primary care is the stuff I like, and I'm pretty sure my career is heading in that direction anyway. But the fact is, the mark of a good primary care doctor is one who can take care not only of the simple things, but who can also recognize more serious, complicated problems and then know what to do about them. If you haven't spent any time with the subspecialists, if you haven't seen what these problems look like, you're not going to be able to recognize them when they present themselves to you in your office. And I resent the fact that this is all being done not to enhance our education, but because it's a financial necessity.

I was really upset about this news the whole day. . . . I think this is only the beginning. In the future, more and more decisions are going to be made that impair our educational experiences, decisions that are made based solely on economic realities. I don't think it's in our best interests, I don't think it's in our patients' best interests, and I don't think it's in the country's best interests. The doctors who are going to serve this country in the future are going to wind up being inadequately trained. Every resident in our program should be very upset about this!

From the tone of Hal's diary, one would think that the entire foundation of the residency program had been shaken by the decision to pull interns and residents from working in some of the subspecialty clinics. In fact, although his statement about the primary motivation for making this change being financial was true, the decision to pull house officers out of the subspecialty clinics was clearly in the best educational interest of the residents. In those clinics, the house officers used to be worked unmercifully; teaching was minimal and service was at a maximum. The learning of subspecialty medicine—the ability to understand and deal with problems such as heart murmurs, diabetes, blood or protein in the urine—comes not from spending two or three afternoons a year in an overcrowded cardiology, endocrinology, or nephrology clinic, but rather during elective rotations in the second and third years of training, periods when an entire month can be devoted to learning the finer points of the subspecialty. But Hal was convinced that a grave injustice was being done to him and his fellow trainees, and for the next two months, he fixated on the problem. On November 12, he said:

I'm feeling really sad. So far, this has been the lowest point of the year for me. Maybe it's because it's getting dark early, maybe it's because I'm so tired all the time, maybe it's because of the changes in our program that we were told about at the intern retreat, but it's really getting to me. I'm very unhappy and concerned about how these changes are going to affect my training. The more I've thought about it, the more I've realized that pulling us from the subspecialty clinics during our OPD rotations is going to make us less effective doctors. . . . I don't know exactly what's going to happen, but I'm very unhappy. This news has killed off my motivation.

As November ended, Hal became increasingly obsessed with the situation. His paranoia that the directors of the program were attempting to sabotage his education led him to seek advice from all sorts of people. As an entry he made in his diary on December 14 indicates, one of those people was Alan Cozza, chief of the pediatric service at Jonas Bronck Hospital during *The Intern Blues*, who has since moved on to become an associate dean of the Schweitzer School of Medicine. Here's that entry:

I'm still quite pissed off about the changes that are scheduled to occur in the residency program next month. I talked to Alan Cozza and explained to him what was going on concerning the subspecialty clinics. He hadn't heard anything about it, but he fully agreed with me and said that he felt that if they keep us out of the subspecialty clinics, it would be a disaster. He advised me to organize the housestaff. That's what I'm going to try to do. But first, I'm going to meet with Richard Andrews and Mike Miller [the two directors of the training program] *to tell them how upset I am and see what they have to say about it. I'm still really upset.*

And from an entry recorded on January 9:

There's still no closure on my concerns about the loss of subspecialty clinic experience. I'm getting the feeling that nobody in the administration wants to deal with this issue. I've been trying desperately to arrange a meeting with the powers that be to get them to have an open meeting with the housestaff about it. Before Christmas week, I met with Mike Miller and told him how upset and angry I was. He said, "Don't worry. I'll come to residents' lunch on the first Friday after New Year's Day and let people know exactly what's happening."

So the first Friday after New Year's Day came. I had just gotten back from vacation, and I asked Mike Miller if he could postpone the meeting for one week, because, having been away myself, I hadn't had a chance to put up any signs or publicize the meeting. He said, "Well, look, it's no big deal. It's just going to be a few minutes. Let's at least get the ball rolling." So I said fine, let's do it. At least some attention was being paid to the problem.

But then it turned out that there was going to be a special infectious disease lecture given at residents' lunch. Dr. Miller told me not to worry about it, that he'd wait until the lecture was over and say what he was going to say.

Fine. So that morning, I busted my hump running around the place, telling everyone to come to residents' lunch, because there was an important issue that was going to be discussed. I managed to get a whole bunch of people to show up, but when I got to the conference room, one of the chief residents told me that Dr. Miller had been called away and wasn't going to be able to make it. He hadn't told the chief resident anything about the issue we had discussed.

To say I was discouraged about this is an understatement. I tried to reschedule the meeting with Dr. Miller, but he told me that he was about to leave on vacation and wouldn't be back for three weeks. I spoke with Richard Andrews, who at least isn't going anywhere. He said he'd be happy to come to residents' lunch to discuss the issue next Friday, but he was already scheduled to be somewhere else that morning, so he couldn't guarantee that he'd be available. So now I don't know what I'm going to do. Everybody seems to be stonewalling about this.

The good part of all this is that I've managed to drum up a lot of interest among the housestaff. I've piqued people's curiosity and they want to know what's going on. Which is good; that's the way it should be.

The proposed meeting with Mike Miller and Richard Andrews never actually occurred. Hal gradually became more depressed by the seeming lack of interest from the people who run the residency program. Simultaneously, he was becoming more overwhelmed by work and exhaustion. As January came to a close, the final ingredient was added to Hal's depression stew: During his final night on call in the emergency room, Hal developed shaking chills, muscle aches, and a sore throat. Using one of the oral thermometers in the ER's nursing triage area, he found that his temperature had soared to 102°. At about 1:00 A.M., while driving home, he recorded a diary entry; the tape reveals a whispering, cracking voice, the result of advancing laryngitis. During the entry, Hal says repeatedly that he feels like shit, that what he really needed was a few days off to recover from this illness, but that he knew this was impossible. The next day, he was scheduled to start a new rotation on the pediatric floor at West Bronx Hospital, the most demanding ward rotation in our system. He was dreading what awaited him. That diary entry ended with these words:

Now I'm home. I'm going to sleep. I've got to be up again at 6:30 to start work at West Bronx. I hope I feel better after a few hours of sleep. God, I really feel like shit.

His next entry was recorded on February 3:

Well [coughing], I never did manage to get up at 6:30 that next morning. I was overtaken with my first illness of the year [coughing]. I got the flu. The fucking flu! One hundred two degree fever, muscle aches, headache, everything. That's what I get for working with all those sick children in the emergency room.

I had to call in sick for the first time. I didn't want to, but when I woke up at 6:15 that next morning to get out of bed, I almost fell over and cracked my skull [coughing]. I felt sick and tired and dehydrated, and I just turned over and went back to sleep. I slept all that morning and afternoon, and then I stayed in bed and eventually slept some more [coughing]. I'm not doing this for effect, I really do have to cough. By that afternoon, I was feeling a little better, and knew I'd be able to get back to work the next day. But by then, I'd lost my voice. I'm better, but I still don't have my voice back.

Anyway, I just spent my first night on call as an intern on Six-A [West Bronx Hospital's Pediatric ward]. *What a fucking hellhole . . . boy oh boy oh boy! The paperwork and the bureaucracy in that place are unbelievable. You're absolutely crushed with crap to fill out. And it's all nothing but crap! [coughing] Uh-oh, I just coughed up some lung cookies.*

Some of the nurses on the floor are pretty good, but most of them are lazy. I mean really lazy! Especially the night nurses. And I can say without reservation that a few of the nurses who were on with me last night are among the dumbest human beings I have ever met. The reason they like working nights is that at night, there's nobody around to look over their shoulders. There are no bosses around, so they know they can get away with bullshit. They cannot do more than one thing at a time, and they have two speeds: slow and stop. And they do jack squat!

On top of that, they're always harassing us over stupid details that have absolutely no clinical significance and absolutely no bearing on the care and management of the patients. They don't have much medical knowledge, so they don't understand why we're doing what we're doing. . . . They don't have any judgment about what's important and what's not. But they sure know how to harass us. They're never shy about calling and saying, "You have to sign this," "You have to do that," "I can't give that without the orders saying this." It's absolutely maddening.

Last night, I spent over an hour and a half arguing with one of the nurses and the nursing supervisor, who's another genius. It all started because I wanted to give a child Ribovarin. The nurse didn't want to give it. I argued and argued with her, because she obviously didn't understand anything about why I was giving it. I just couldn't get her to understand. Then she called down her supervisor, and I had to start at the beginning and argue with her all over again.

Finally, in the end, they caved in. At about three in the morning, the medication was finally started. About an hour later, the nurse started giving me grief again about why I'd refused to draw blood cultures before starting the medication. I said to her, for the fiftieth time, "What the hell are you talking about? There are no blood cultures for RSV! We test for RSV by sticking a swab in the kid's nose. I don't have the swab. It's in the virology lab, which will not be open until the morning. That's it. End of story. No more discussion." What a waste of time!

While making this entry, Hal, his voice still hoarse from laryngitis, was actually yelling into the tape recorder. A few days later, on February 8, he recorded his next entry. In this entry, Hal's voice sounded different, distant and very soft and sad. I didn't listen to this tape until months later when I was working on the transcription, but had I heard it at the time it was occurring, I would have driven to Hal's apartment, picked him up, and brought him to the psychiatric emergency room. Here's the entry:

I don't think I've ever been more unhappy than I am right now [coughing]. *This ward is fucking unbelievable! The place is overwhelming. I'm currently carrying fifteen patients, and I don't know how I'm supposed to keep up with any of them. There are so many things I'm supposed to do, so much paperwork, so much scut. It's too much for me. It just doesn't seem to make any sense.*

Most of my patients are just asthmatics, but some of them are much more complicated [coughing]. *The load is starting to crush me. I feel like I'm out of control, foundering, and I'm afraid there's going to be a disaster. I'm frightened, I'm not getting enough supervision, and I don't know what to look for. Something bad is bound to happen in a situation like this.*

Today I had a problem with one of my patients simply because I misread the chart. The nurse's note in the chart said that the baby was having diarrheal stools. I couldn't read the part that said "diarrheal" and thought it just said that she was just having stools, which is normal. I got the bloodwork back late last night and found that her bicarb was down to 8 [bicarbonate level in the blood should be at least 20; a low bicarbonate level occurs in conditions that result in acidosis; in this child, the ongoing diarrhea was the source of the low bicarb]. *The fact that it was abnormal surprised me, because I couldn't see any reason for it being low.*

So I knew the bicarb was low, but I didn't get a chance to repeat the test last night. I was so overwhelmed with admissions and other stuff that I just couldn't get to it. This morning on rounds, our resident, Kathy Firestone, took a look at the baby and said, "This kid looks sick." Sure enough, she'd been having diarrhea all through the night and was now so dehydrated that she needed an immediate injection of normal saline solution to prevent her from going into shock. Thank God Kathy was able to get an IV into her; I sure as hell wouldn't have been able to do it. We gave the baby some fluid and that seems to have turned her around.

But the fact that we fixed her is not the point. The point is, she got that sick because I screwed up. I hadn't been paying attention. That's terrible.

I was feeling so low this afternoon that I went to have a talk with Peter Chang [one of the chief residents]. He was nice to me, and he looked into the situation immediately, which was nice, but he wound up blaming Kathy for not supervising me closely enough. He told her she should have figured out sooner that the baby was that sick. Kathy got angry, and I felt even worse, because not only had I screwed up, but now she was getting blamed for it. I mean, after all, she was really the one who saved us today.

I just don't know how I can go on with this sort of existence. I'm trying my best, but it's not good enough. I'm not being well supervised, and I have a ton of stuff to do. I'm post-call, it's 3:00 P.M., and I can't stand being here anymore. Even though there's still so much work to do, I've decided to just go home and get some sleep. I feel as if I've left so much to do for tomorrow and the next day, things that I'm not doing. . . . I feel as if I'll never be able to catch up. I wasn't able to write a note on one of my patients yesterday. I didn't have time to write notes on three patients today. The work just gets thicker and thicker, and the farther behind you get, the farther behind you get. It's so pointless coming to work, I just don't know why I should go on like this.

I'm really not happy. Right now, I feel so unhappy, I feel like going home and crying. I don't know how anybody can stand this, and I don't know if I'm par for the course, or if other interns are having an easier time. My friend Fran, who's an intern on the other team, she looks like she's having a cake-walk through this place.

Maybe I feel so bad because I'm post-call and everything seems so dire. But I've been post-call before and I haven't ever felt this bad. I don't know. I just don't have an answer.

I used to think that doing all these admissions and working hard would build character. Right now, I feel as if it builds frustration and hatred. I feel just so miserable; so miserable.

I'm on call again Saturday. I hope I can survive it. I hope I can make it to Sunday, when I'll be able to get some sleep. Oh God.

Hal's February 8 entry represented his absolute lowest point of the year. Thankfully, things quickly improved from here. By the time he recorded his next diary entry on February 9, his mood had begun to lighten, at least a little.

Today was a little better. We got a handle on that baby who got so sick, the one whose bicarb was so low. It looks as if she was septic [had a bacterial infection in her blood]. We started her on antibiotics, and it looks like she's responding to them. So at least that's a relief.

The other thing is I managed to get some of the discharge paperwork out of the way and to set myself up for tomorrow. The really big help, though, was that Kathy, our resident, redistributed the patients and I was able to give three away. I had fifteen patients when I came to work today. That's just way too many for any one person to manage. I gave three away and discharged two, so now I'm down to ten. Still not great, but a lot more manageable.

Last night, when I reached home, I walked through the door and just started to cry. I burst into tears and told my wife, "I don't want to do this anymore. I don't want to be a doctor." I felt so overwhelmed and lost that I just didn't know what to make of things. I didn't know how I was possibly going to get up this morning, get my clothes on, get to work, and get through the day.

Robin just hugged me. Eventually, she took me into the bedroom, helped me take off my clothes, and got into bed. She brought me some soup, and after eating it, I just fell asleep. I don't know what I would have done if Robin hadn't been there last night. I'm afraid to think. . . .

But I feel better today. I think I'm starting to get on top of things again. I have my discharges all set for tomorrow; I'm going to take some paperwork home tonight and try to get my discharges done for the next day. If I can finish those, all I'll have to do tomorrow is write my progress notes and that'll be it. . . . So things are definitely starting to come under control. So that's the story. I'm just trying to work things out.

By the next night, Hal seemed to have climbed back on his feet:

And today was a little bit better than yesterday. My service has undergone a major diuresis: I managed to discharge six patients today. I got the discharges done, I got my notes written, I made plans on all the kids who are staying. Oh man, I feel as if I'm back on top of things again. I'm headed home for dinner now. Unfortunately, I've got to come back tomorrow morning to be on call again. We've cleared out about eleven beds, so the ward's going to be wide open tomorrow. I'm getting ready for another one of those typical ten-admission nights.

Hal's situation continued to improve through much of the rest of the month. He still had some bad nights on call, continued to get into petty arguments with the night nurses, but his state of mind improved day by day. He clearly recognized how bad his life had been, how close to the edge he'd crept. Here's an excerpt from his last entry of the month:

I finally finished my month on Six-A. Just leaving the floor, I felt this huge weight lift off my shoulders. The first minute off the ward, I realized what a stupid, stupid place West Bronx is! Ugh, the bullshit and the paperwork and the bureaucracy and the stupidity is unbelievable. I'm just so glad this month is over. . . .

Having made it through this horrible month, I'm sitting here thinking I'm going to be able to survive my internship. There's no question that over the past few months, I've had some serious, serious doubts, but now, having made it through a month on Six-A, I know I'll be able to survive anything. And there are only four months to go. I definitely think this was a turning point for me.

In the last four days, I've been on call twice and post-call twice. I covered for my friend, Fran, last night. She started her vacation today and needed to be off last night so she could catch a flight to the Bahamas. I volunteered to cover for her, which pushed me to every other call. It's caused me to feel really blitzed, really out of it, but to be honest, I don't give a shit. I'm finished with Six-A, and I never have to be an intern up there again!

Hal's response to surviving February is not unique. February is a turning point. In March, the light magically begins to appear at the end of the tunnel. After February, the worst is clearly over.

9

M A R C H

The Ninth Rotation:
Match Day—A Light Appears
at the End of the Tunnel

So February, the worst month in the year for interns, is the turning point. February is miserable, but the misery of February serves a purpose: It makes the relief that comes in March that much sweeter.

Ah, March, the month during which spring starts, the last full season of internship! Sunlight returns in March. The days grow longer, and for the first time since October, house officers (as well as everyone else in the Northeast) leave work while the streets are still light, getting home before the sun goes down.

In late March in New York, the temperature climbs into the higher thirties and forties. For the first time since December, the hard-packed gray, cruddy snow that's covered the ground like a straitjacket melts away, allowing the grass and trees to come to life. As the danger associated with patches of black ice fades, people can once again set foot without trepidation on the sidewalks and streets.

But by far the most important factor bringing smiles back to the faces of burned-out interns is an event that occurs every year on the third Wednesday of March. On that afternoon, during the annual Resident Match Day event, fourth-year medical students throughout the United States find out where they'll be working as interns beginning July 1.

Match Day is one of those bizarre, sadistic rituals that could only have been invented by some high-ranking official in medical education. Unfortunately for those who are forced to participate, the event has changed very little since it was invented in the 1970s as a way of preventing highly competitive residency programs from exerting an unfair advantage on senior medical students. As such, the experience I survived back in 1979 is comparable to the experience of students today.

At the beginning of March of my senior year, my classmates and I were sent an official notice, signed by our school's dean of academic affairs, ordering us to report to the lecture hall on Wednesday, March 15 at precisely 1:00 P.M. Each of us knew about Match Day: We'd heard frightening stories from the interns with whom we'd worked since beginning our third-year rotations, and we hadn't liked what we'd heard. As we waited for the day to arrive, my friends and I remained quiet, never actually discussing the event or its implications out loud.

When that Wednesday finally arrived, members of our class nervously assembled back in the lecture hall where we'd spent so much time three years before. Without even thinking, we each took the exact seat we'd occupied every day as first-year students. Being at ease was important on Match Day; this was one stressful event.

The reason for the tension was rooted in our knowledge of the official and sacred regulations that govern Match Day. In most professions, finding a new job is a straightforward process. A person interested in a particular job fills out an application and is invited for an interview. If during that interview the applicant makes a positive impression, and if his credentials are good enough, someone in management will offer him the position. Following the tendering of the job offer, based on a number of factors that include salary and the benefits package being offered, the applicant has the right either to accept the job and begin work or reject it and begin the search for another position. But this simple system, which has been good enough for American business for decades, is apparently much too simple to work when the job being offered is an internship slot. Clearly, another system, one more byzantinely bureaucratic and inhumane, had to be developed for offering jobs to medical school graduates.

The way Match Day works sounds simple. In January of his senior year, after interviewing at all the programs to which he has applied, the medical student submits a list of those programs, ranked from first to last choice, to the National Residency Matching Program (NRMP). Simultaneously, each of the teaching hospitals throughout the United States that maintains residency programs submits a list of all senior medical students who have applied for positions. These programs similarly rank the applicants from most to least desirable. Once these lists are received, all the information is fed into NRMP's computer and the machine couples applicants and programs, thus creating the Match.

One might think this matching procedure would play itself out uneventfully: First, a simple letter originating from NRMP Central would be sent out; after receiving that letter in the mail a few days later, the senior medical student would fill out a form, checking off a box before one of these two choices: "Yes, I accept your internship position" or "No, I'd rather burn in hell for all of eternity than spend a single day working in your hellhole of a hospital." He'd return the form and life would simply proceed from there.

Instead, the results of the computer's match are printed, wrapped in envelopes, and stored in impenetrable secret vaults at NRMP Central for two excruciatingly long months. Finally, on the third Wednesday in March, the results are released simultaneously to medical schools and the residency programs. On that afternoon, all across the United States, senior medical students assemble in large lecture halls and the envelopes bearing their hospital assignments for the next year are distributed slowly, agonizingly, one by one. At more than 100 American medical schools, the process is exactly the same: A name is called and the student rises and tentatively stumbles toward the front of the room. With the rest of his class looking on, the envelope is handed to him by the person, usually a dean, entrusted with maintaining the "sanctity" of the Match. The envelope is cautiously opened, and the student either sighs a sigh of great relief, because he's matched at one of his top choices and his dreams have been fulfilled, or lapses into an immediate and terrifying anxiety attack, because he's gotten his third or fourth or, God forbid, his fifth or sixth choice, and has immediately come to the conclusion that his life has been permanently ruined.

These anxiety attacks are fueled by a very important fact that is known to all subscribers of the Match. Unlike normal job offers, the Match assignments are unconditionally and irrevocably binding. Unless there are extraordinarily extenuating circumstances, such as death or, potentially, a disabling illness, there is no chance of transferring to another program once an assignment to a hospital has been made. Once the internship assignment is made, both the hospital and the young doctor are locked in, at least for one year. So back on March 15, 1979, as our dean of academic affairs entered the hall, took his place at the podium, and, without any introductory remarks, began calling off the names of my classmates in random order, I prayed that my dreams would be realized, that, when I tore open the flap of my envelope, the name printed on the sheet inside would be the Children's Hospital of Philadelphia, the program I'd listed as the number one choice on my Match list.

Sitting in the lecture hall, my personal hell lasted until the names of nearly three-quarters of my classmates had been called. As I sat in my comfortable old seat, watching each individual drama play itself out at the front of the lecture hall, my anxiety level increased with each passing minute. Finally, my name was called. I rose from my seat and walked carefully to the front of the auditorium. I was handed the envelope and cautiously tore open its flap. My spirits sank when I saw the words "Boston Medical Center—Pediatrics" on the paper that filled that envelope.

The Boston Medical Center's pediatric program not only hadn't been my first choice, it hadn't even been my second choice. During the previous fall, when I visited the five programs I ultimately ranked, there had been something about the Medical Center, some feeling I couldn't exactly put my finger on, that bothered me. No one I spoke with expressed any misgivings about the program; everyone, attending physicians, interns, and residents, seemed satisfied with the place, but there was something, an undercurrent of tension that I sensed. This feeling had ultimately caused me to place the program below two others (Children's Hospital of Philadelphia and Massachusetts General Hospital) on my final rank list.

It wasn't until the next fall that I came to understand what that certain unrest I'd sensed the year before actually was. As an intern who was unhappy with the training program, I wanted to make sure I had access to intern applicants; in an attempt to help them avoid making the same mistake I'd made, I wanted to tell them of my experiences. But during the week before internship interviews began, I received a memo from the chief resident advising me to stay far away from visiting applicants or else. Although it was not stated, the implication was that if I frightened off unsuspecting applicants, my on-call schedule for the remainder of the year would suffer. And then I realized why everyone I'd spoken with the year before had seemed satisfied: The program directors had identified and taken steps to silence anyone who was unhappy.

Initially, I'd planned to disregard the chief resident's advice; there was something important at stake here. But the more I thought about it, the less desire I had to make waves; after all, an extra night on call was something to be avoided at all costs.

Of course, as I stood at the front of the auditorium in the Bronx with the Match letter in my hand, I didn't know any of this. Trying to keep myself from crying right there in front of my classmates, I quickly walked up the steps and left the lecture hall as rapidly as I could, trying to come to grips with the fact that I would be spending at least the coming year (and possibly two years in addition to that) at my third-choice program. Oh man, the Boston Medical Center; I needed a drink!

Although Match Day may be psychic hell for the fourth-year medical students whose future existences are systematically toyed with, the event is a cause for wild celebration to the tired interns who slowly emerge from the shells of their late-winter depressions. On Match Day afternoon at residency programs around the country, a single sheet of paper is pinned up on a corner of the bulletin board on which the monthly house-staff on-call schedules are usually posted. Almost immediately, a crowd of interns gathers around this sheet. Each intern reads the contents of the sheet and begins to smile. That sheet, of course, bears the names of the fourth-year medical students who have matched to that program. The interns understand that these are their replacements, the unfortunate putzes who, come July 1, will step into their shoes and become the scut dogs of the future. Suddenly, the interns realize that the end is definitely in sight.

Hal Burkins, who was as low as anyone I've ever seen during February, celebrated Match Day by throwing a party. Although it wasn't officially Match Day he was celebrating (the day also happened to be his thirtieth birthday), just knowing that, after so long, there was now an actual name for the person who would take his place on the on-call schedule in a few short months made the celebration of this milestone much sweeter.

Hal's wife, Robin, who planned the celebration, had invited the entire intern group and their significant others. Because a quarter of the interns were on call that night and another quarter were post-call and therefore exhausted, only about thirty people managed to actually make it to their apartment. But thirty people were more than enough to celebrate the double occasion. The celebrants danced, ate, and drank until after two in the morning. Although I didn't attend, I was told afterward that everyone had a terrific time.

Hal's buoyancy during March was also helped by the fact
that he spent the month working in the outpatient department
at Mt. Scopus Medical Center. Here's some of his diary entry of
March 23:

I really enjoy the OPD [outpatient department]. *There isn't all
the drudgery that's involved in managing patients on the inpatient units. You don't have to track down every lab result or write
silly progress notes on every patient every day. You just show up
at the clinic or the emergency room, see the patients who are scheduled to be seen, figure out what's going on with them, treat the
problem, and either send them home or admit them to the ward.
It's simple, it's straightforward, and there's no bullshit involved.
It's sort of bad that you never get follow-up on any of the patients,
that you never find out what actually happened to any of them,
but on the other hand, it's not the tense, labor-intensive work
that's involved when you're working on the wards.*

*So life has been a lot more relaxing. In the morning, I don't have
to be at work until 8:00 A.M., so I can sleep a little later. When I'm
on call, I get to come home as soon as my shift ends, so I never
have to sleep in the hospital. It's heaven. What could be better?*

*Today, I spent the day in two subspecialty clinics. I loved it.
These are the same clinics that are being eliminated from our
schedule next year when the new rules go into effect. It appears as
if they're not going to change this decision, and I am still not
happy about it. It's going to happen next July: We're going to be
separated from these clinics, and we're never going to have a
chance to learn how to handle these specific problems. I'm not
happy about it, but I don't have any recourse. I'm stuck.*

*Anyway this morning, I went to endocrine clinic and in the
afternoon, I was in hematology clinic. They were both pretty good.
I saw three patients in each clinic, saw some things I've never seen*

before, and learned some things. That's the way it's supposed to be for interns and residents.

The month also allowed Hal to gain insights into the changes that had occurred since the beginning of the academic year, especially how his internship had affected his relationship with patients and their families. On March 30, in his last diary entry of the month, he said:

One thing that's happening to me that I don't like is that I find myself getting impatient and frustrated and even angry at parents who come to the clinics or the emergency room and don't speak a word of English. They bring their child to the doctor for a checkup, because they have a question about something, and they can't communicate that question or even give a history to the doctors who are trying to help them. They come into the office and sit there, waiting for me to go and find someone who will translate for them. And really, I try to be tolerant about it, but this is becoming very frustrating. Now, I'd love to learn Spanish and I know it must sound racist, but these people come to New York, they live in our country, a country where English is still the official language, and I think they should at least make the effort to help us help them.

Another thing that's beginning to bother me a lot is that parents will bring their child into the emergency room, and I'll ask them what medication the child is on, and they'll say, "Oh, I don't know. Some pink stuff." Now that really blows my mind. Your child is taking medication. You're coming to the hospital for some help, you're being seen by a doctor, and you don't even know the name of the medication your child is taking? That's insane!

I try not to lose my temper or show my frustration with these people, but it's really starting to piss me off. I tell them as calmly as I can that you really have to know the name of the medication your child is on, that it is irresponsible of them as a parent not to know this information. It's irritating, and it makes me feel impatient and burned out. We're trying to help them, but the patient has to take some of the responsibility. It's as simple as that.

It's good to have gotten that off my chest. Most of the parents we see are really very good. They're concerned about their children, they take responsibility, and they do everything appropriately. It's only a small minority who piss me off, but the effect of that small minority goes a long way to counterbalancing the good feelings you get from taking care of the responsible ones.

The combination of Match Day, the longer periods of sunlight, the warmer weather, and his rotation in the outpatient department went a long way toward bringing Hal Burkins back from the ledge on which he was poised. And during the first two weeks of April, he went on vacation.

10

A P R I L

The Tenth Rotation:
Interns on Vacation

I finish in the OPD next week and then I go on vacation. Carole and I have decided to go to Cancún. We were thinking about going back to that hotel in the Poconos we went to during my last vacation, but Carole thought I'd been tortured enough for one lifetime . . . I still think that maybe we should go. I mean, if I go someplace nice and actually have a good time, how am I going to be able to come back to the Bronx to finish the last couple of months of this wonderful experience?
    Mark Greenberg, M.D., prior to his final vacation

Like most other things, interns approach planning for their vacations differently than other people. These too small islands of downtime are not just an opportunity to get away from the realities of life for a few days and relax, they are critically important to the intern's survival. Having had so little time during their workweek to perform normal activities, house officers wind up putting enormous pressure on themselves to get done such mundane tasks as visiting their parents, completing their tax returns, washing and drying their clothes, cleaning their apartment, eating dinner, and having some semblance of a normal social life during their holidays. Simultaneously, interns and residents understand that they must catch up on some of the weeks and weeks worth of sleep they've missed during the preceding months. In trying to accomplish everything, in attempting to crowd all of this into the one or two weeks they have off, house officers often wind up ruining their vacations and having a miserable time.

Probably the best description of a typically manic intern vacation from hell was given by Mark Greenberg after he returned from his first vacation (a quote just prior to his second vacation appears above). Here's a portion of Mark's diary entry from *The Intern Blues* dated October 4, 1985:

My vacation wasn't exactly what I'd call wonderful. No, wonderful is definitely not the word I'd use. How would I describe it? What word would I use? Lousy. Lousy is definitely the word I'd use. Lousy bordering on shitty.

The vacation started off with my brother and me in my car, driving south as fast as we could. We didn't have any real endpoint in mind. I just needed to get out of New York. I was trying to find a place where cockroaches don't exist. Actually, that's not exactly true. We were heading for Cincinnati. We both have friends there who we haven't seen for a long time, and we decided to go visit them. Yes, there's nothing more romantic or restful than driving a thousand miles and spending a week with your younger brother visiting friends in Cincinnati in late September. The whole experience almost made the Bronx seem nice. Almost . . .

Okay, so it wasn't romantic, but Carole [Mark's then girlfriend and future wife] and I sure made up for that in the second week of my vacation. We went to the romance capital of the East, Pocono Castle, a resort hotel catering to the honeymoon crowd. What a place! I knew we had made a mistake when the first thing the bellboy showed us was the heart-shaped bathtub in our room. Carole said she liked it; I thought I showed great restraint by keeping myself from puking right there on the spot.

But that was far from the worst of it. We went down to the dining room that first night and discovered that everybody, every last couple, was there on their honeymoon. It was Carole and me and four hundred newlyweds! The place was disgusting; the food was horrible, the decorating job was ostentatious, the rooms were dirty, and it rained all week. All for two hundred bucks a day! Just the kind of relaxing environment I needed.

In the dining room, they put us at a table with another couple. These two were great: They had just been remarried for the second time. They were reformed drug addicts. We spent every meal chatting about AIDS!

Although Mark complained, he undoubtedly would have been more pissed off had he finished medical school twenty years earlier. Like the eighty-hour workweek, a reasonable salary, and health benefits, vacation time is a relatively new development for house officers. Prior to the 1970s, interns and residents worked for fifty-two straight weeks without more than a weekend off.

The experience of my father-in-law was typical. After graduating from medical school in New York in early June 1952, he and my future mother-in-law, who was then two months pregnant with my future wife, Beth, climbed into their beat-up Oldsmobile with all their possessions and drove to California. In less than a week, they found an apartment, moved in, and got settled as best they could. On July 1, my father-in-law began his rotating internship (so called because he spent the year rotating through each of the important specialty services, spending four months in internal medicine, five months in surgery, two months in pediatrics, and one month in OB/GYN) at Cedars of Lebanon Hospital in Los Angeles. For the next twelve months, he worked fifty-two straight 110-hour weeks.

Although the work was hard and demanding, neither my mother-in-law nor my father-in-law seemed to question the lack of vacation time. "Going away anywhere was out of the question," my mother-in-law told me. "Jerry was being paid a salary of fifty dollars a month. On that, we couldn't even afford to go out to a movie! There was no way we could have afforded to go away on vacation."

Life became a little more complicated for my future in-laws at the end of his internship year. Having accepted a residency position in orthopedic surgery back in New York, my father-in-law was expected to show up for his first day of work on July 1, 1953. Now, it's kind of difficult to be on call in Los Angeles on the night of June 30, move a wife, baby, and an apartment's worth of furniture and possessions three thousand miles, and show up fresh and ready to begin work in a new program on July 1. He had to beg permission to take a week's leave (without pay, of course) from his new job in order to give him the time to drive cross-country, locate a new apartment, and get settled in. They made it, and a week after he'd ended his job in LA, he began his residency tired, disoriented, and more than a little out of sorts.

Dr. X, who trained in California in the early 1960s, had a similar experience. In the postscript of his book *Intern*, Dr. X, who had just completed internal medicine, the final rotation of his internship, wrote:

During those last few days [of internship], I remember that Ann [Dr. X's wife] and I had thoughts for only one thing: a rest and vacation. I had a grandiose dream of doing nothing but eating and sleeping for a solid week (I still have the same dream, still unfulfilled). Ann read travel folders and figured how we could manage a week on the beach in Baja California for practically no money at all. Neither of us got our way, because state licensure exams faced me just three weeks off. I did not sleep and we did not travel. I studied. . . .

Spurred on by the newly organized Committee of Interns and Residents—the house officer's union—the movement to reform the conditions under which the housestaff worked proceeded slowly through the 1960s and 1970s. Thankfully, when I started my training, the holiday situation had changed for the better. Built into my internship schedule at the Boston Medical Center, I was fortunate enough to have three weeks off. I was not free to choose when I would take those vacations; they were awarded to me in one-week blocks, assigned randomly during each of my three rotations in the hospital's outpatient department.

Today, I have absolutely no recollection of either of my first two weeks of vacation. But I remember the third week as if it were yesterday. It occurred in late April, and by then what I needed more than anything else was to get out of Boston. I was exhausted, pissed off at the entire world, and, to make matters worse, spring was taking its sweet time getting to New England. Boston was still frigid and, unbelievably, there was still a thin sheet of snow clinging to the ground. I understood that spending a few days lying on the beach in some sun-soaked tropical island paradise drinking piña coladas wasn't going to solve all my problems, but, on the other hand, it clearly wasn't going to do me any harm, either.

As was the case with my in-laws during my father-in-law's internship and Dr. X during his, a check of our finances revealed that, unless we were suddenly to come into an inheritance, there wasn't much of a chance we could make it anywhere near that Caribbean island. By that point in the year, we were practically broke. Our money problems resulted from two facts: First, as an intern, I was getting paid a salary of $15,000 for the year, a lot more than house officers in my father-in-law's era had been paid, but still a sum that, when you considered the number of hours I'd been working, translated to a wage of roughly $2.50 per hour; second, Beth, who'd been living and working in New York during the first half of that year, had spent much of our spare cash flying the shuttle round-trip between our two cities every weekend. As a result, we were nearly broke and we didn't have enough money to fly round-trip to Bangor, Maine, let alone to the Bahamas.

So on the Friday night that my vacation actually began, rather than packing up our bathing suits and sunblock, Beth and I sat at our kitchen table, glaring at each other, discussing over and over again our not-very-tempting options. After about an hour of arguing, Beth finally said, "Why don't we just get into the car, start driving south, and keep on driving until we hit warm weather?" Realizing that this was the only option that made any sense, I agreed. And so, early the next morning, we loaded our stuff into our car and headed for the Mass Pike.

It looked as if for the first time that entire year, we might have actually lucked out. Although New England was still frigid, summer had arrived earlier than usual in the Middle Atlantic states. By the time we hit the Connecticut-New York border at around noon that Saturday, the temperature had climbed into the mid-sixties. We kept on driving until late after-noon, when we hit the resort town of Wildwood on the New Jersey shore. Tired, but happy with our surroundings, we decided that we'd reached our destination.

Our week in Wildwood was sensational. The weather was perfect every day, the sky continuously cloudless, and the sun warm and bright. Each afternoon, the temperature rose into the eighties. Because it was still April, the beach, boardwalk, hotels, and restaurants were all nearly deserted. Except for the seabirds and the few natives, we had the place essentially all to our-selves. We slept until eleven o'clock each morning, laid out on the beach all afternoon, and ate in cheap restaurants every night. By our fourth day at the shore, I actually began to feel some semblance of my old, pre-intern self returning.

Because of our lack of money, Beth and I were forced to keep to a strict budget. Even though we were helped immensely by the fact that, it being off-season, the price of everything, includ-ing our motel room and meals, was unbelievably low, by the end of the week, we were pretty much tapped out. Before leav-ing our motel early Sunday morning for the return trip to Boston, we checked our wallets: Combining our resources, we had exactly nineteen dollars left. We figured that if we charged the gas on our Mobil credit card and put aside ten dollars for tolls, we'd have just enough for lunch at McDonald's. But it was going to be awfully close.

Back in the car, we began to head north along the Garden State Parkway, a trip that, under the best of circumstances, would last at least eight hours, and, what with Sunday traffic, would probably take a whole lot longer. I was searching for some distraction to take our minds off the brutal trip ahead, and so when Beth announced that she needed to take a bathroom break just as I was approaching the exit ramp for the Atlantic

City Expressway, I used the opportunity to get off the highway.

At that time, Atlantic City was undergoing its major transition. The year before, the city council had voted to legalize gambling, and Caesar's Palace, the first of the gargantuan casinos, had only recently opened. Since Beth, who has always been opposed to gambling in any form, had never actually seen the inside of a casino, I figured this would be a great opportunity to educate her.

Beth wasn't happy with this decision. During the short trip along the Atlantic City Expressway, she argued and yelled. She did not, under any circumstances, want to set foot into any such "den of iniquity," as she referred to the casino. But by then, she *really* needed to use a bathroom and so wasn't in a position to put up much of a fight. After reaching downtown, I parked along a side street and we just about ran the block and a half to the entrance of the hotel. After using the facilities, Beth reluctantly let me take her hand and drag her toward the glittering casino. "I'm only letting you do this because I know you have absolutely no money left to blow," she said.

At that time, I believed I was quite an expert in casino gambling. As the son of parents who loved to bet on just about anything, I'd visited a lot of casinos since turning eighteen. So with me as the guide and Beth reluctantly and only halfheartedly following behind, we entered the casino. "These are the slot machines," I told her as we passed the rows of slot machines. "These are the crap tables," I added as we passed the crap tables. "Here are the one-dollar blackjack tables. . . . Here are the five-dollar blackjack tables. . . . And here . . . is my mother!"

Yes, miraculously, unexpectedly, perched on a stool, hunching over what appeared to be an enormous pile of multicolored chips at one of the crowded five-dollar blackjack tables, sat my own mother! Momentarily stunned by this revelation, my body soon filled with a warm, comfortable feeling. My mother! I hadn't seen either of my parents for more than five months, not since we'd had Thanksgiving dinner together at my aunt's apartment in Queens. And here she was, sitting not five feet away from me, doubling down after drawing a pair of aces.

I stood silently at that distance for a few seconds, watching as the dealer covered one of my mother's aces with a queen of diamonds and the other with a ten of spades. "Yes!" my mother yelled in exultation, her left hand clenching into a fist that she raised over her head.

"Mom," I shouted in response, now approaching closer and tapping her on the shoulder.

She turned her head slightly, catching my presence out of the corner of her eye. "Bob," she said, seeming slightly confused. "What are you doing here?"

"I had vacation this week, remember? We're on our way back to Boston from the shore. We just stopped off for a minute. What a surprise!"

As I was saying these words, the dealer matched the two stacks of chips laid out on the table in front of my mother's seat with two identical stacks. Mom turned away from me to rake in her winnings and to settle on her bet for the next hand. "Look, Bob," she said as I bent to kiss her cheek, "I really can't talk now. I'm on a roll." She gestured to all the multicolored chips that had grown in number even while we'd been watching. "Here, take these," she continued, handing me four twenty-five dollar chips. "Go and have a good time, and we'll talk later."

Beth, who hadn't said a word during this entire encounter, watched me walk away in the direction of the one-dollar blackjack tables. "What do you think you're doing?" she shouted after me.

"Weren't you listening?" I asked. "My mother just gave us

these chips and told us to go have a good time. That's what I'm planning to do: I'm going to play blackjack."

"Let me get this straight," she responded, walking after me. "We're two hundred miles from home, we have less than twenty dollars to our name that has to last until you get your paycheck tomorrow, you were just handed a hundred dollars in cash, and you're going to lose it playing blackjack?" After I'd stared back at her silently with a questioning look on my face for a few seconds, she finally continued: "Bob, don't be a schmuck! Cash in those chips and let's get the hell out of here."

I kept staring at her with that questioning look, but I guess I ultimately realized she was right. When another few seconds had passed and I still hadn't moved, Beth suddenly took me by the hand and led me over to the cashier's cage. "We'd like to cash in," she said, forcing the four chips from my hot little hand and passing them through the opening in the grating. In no time at all, she had been handed five crisp twenty-dollar bills. "Now go and tell your mother we have to hit the road," she continued, pointing me back in the direction of the blackjack table.

I reached my mother just as she had drawn an eight of hearts while holding a seven of diamonds and a six of clubs. "Mom, we've got to go," I said, as the dealer paid her off once again. "It's a long trip back to Boston."

"All right," she replied, not sounding all that disappointed as she simultaneously raked in the additional chips and offered her left cheek for me to kiss. "Drive carefully."

Within ten minutes, we were back on the road. We had lunch that afternoon not at a roadside McDonald's, but at a nice restaurant off I-95 in Connecticut. We made it to Boston in time for dinner at our favorite restaurant in Chinatown. And the next day, my vacation now nothing more than a pleasant memory, I was back in the trenches.

Since my internship ended, I haven't been much of a gambler. I guess my training helped teach me that it often isn't such a good idea to take big risks. But even when I have gambled, I've never again had the success I had on that last day of my vacation at the Jersey shore. And on that day, I didn't even have to place a bet.

The vacations taken by the interns I followed during 1994 and 1995 were not that different from the ones taken nearly ten years earlier by the interns profiled in *The Intern Blues*. Like me, Denise Powers had a vacation in the spring. Also like me, she desperately needed to get away from home, checked her finances and found them to be wanting, and wound up spending time at the Jersey shore. Unfortunately, she made something of a tactical error in choosing her companion. Here are two of Denise's diary entries from early June, 1995:

Saturday, June 10

I don't know what time it is and, to tell you the truth, I don't really care! I'm on vacation! I've been on vacation since last Wednesday, and so far it's been great. I can't even remember what the hell I did on Wednesday. I slept late, I remember that much. And I spent the night out with some friends from home. I was out all night and I did some drinking, and when I got home, I had a king-sized headache.

I've spent the last three days trying to get everything I've been putting off for the last six months done. Like my laundry. I actually went and did my laundry yesterday. It'd been so long since I last washed my clothes, they'd started standing up in the closet by themselves. It was getting pretty disgusting, but what was I supposed to do? I barely had enough time to get to sleep most days; I wasn't going to waste what time I had doing something as worthless as washing my clothes.

I also did a whole bunch of errands that have needed to be done for months. And I cleaned my apartment. Things were really disgusting around here, and I finally started to get things organized.

Now I'm packing. I've been looking forward to this vacation for a long time, trying to figure out where I should go. For a while, I thought about going to New Orleans. One of my friends from med school was supposed to have vacation next week, and we were going to go down there together. But then I looked into how much it was going to cost and I realized I couldn't afford it, and then somebody in her program got sick and they had to change her vacation time, anyway, so that fell through. I was talking to my mother about it, and she suggested that we take a trip down to Atlantic City together for a week. I haven't spent a lot of time with my mother lately (hell, I haven't spent a lot of time with anybody lately), and the price seemed right, so that's what we're going to do. We're going to take the bus down tomorrow and come back on Thursday. Hopefully, it'll be warm and I'll be able to get some sun and hang out on the boardwalk.

I went to the hospital yesterday to pick up my paycheck and decided to stop by the adolescent unit [the ward at Mt. Scopus on which Denise had been working prior to the start of her vacation]. I promised one of my patients I'd come and visit him. It was funny, walking on the ward wearing shorts and a T-shirt. I wish I could have lined up every single nurse I couldn't stand and say, "Ha ha, you have to work today and I don't." I didn't though. I've become very mature about these things.

Anyway, I can't wait to get out of here. AC, here I come!

Tuesday, June 20—11:15 P.M.

About ready to go to bed. Last day of vacation. As usual, I've only managed to do about a third of the things I was planning on doing during these two weeks off. I just can't win.

My trip to Atlantic City was a mistake I hope never to make again. I learned one thing during the trip: My mom and I can no longer take vacations together. No, no, never again! I guess the simplest way to explain it is that we grate on each other's nerves. It was not a lot of fun.

The problem was, all I wanted to do was go down there, get some fresh air, lie on the beach, walk on the boardwalk, get some sleep, and just generally relax. Mom, however, had a whole other agenda. She wanted to party. She wanted to go out to shows, she wanted to see some nightlife, and she refused to do any of this unless I went along with her. Which was something I didn't want to do!

We kept getting into fights. She'd say she wanted to get dressed up and go out and I'd say, "No, Ma, I want to stay in tonight, I'm tired." Then she'd start in with, "What's wrong with you, girl? You used to have some life in you. Where did all that go?" I've tried to explain to her what my life has been like all year, but she just doesn't understand. I guess it's impossible to really understand unless you're living it. And I wouldn't recommend anybody live it.

Anyway, so we fought all week, and the trip was pretty much a disaster. I did manage to get some fresh air and sun, though, so that was pretty good.

Her diary entries during this vacation illustrate some of the changes that occurred to Denise during her internship. Having started the year headstrong, street-smart, and full of energy, Denise was willing to take on attending physicians, like Erica Cintron, or anyone else who got in her way, ready to go out and party even after the worst on-call night. But as the year wore on and the work started to grind her down, Denise's words began to reflect a growing fatigue and weariness of the spirit. At first, this was seen in her need to go right home on post-call days and get right into bed. Later, as seen in these vacation entries, she became so weary she couldn't even keep up with her middle-aged mother. The liveliness with which she'd begun the year, the ebullience that so characterized the preintern Denise, had been beaten out of her.

These diary entries also demonstrate the change that occurred in the relationship between Denise and her mother. All through her internship, Denise had come to depend on her friends and family. Her mother had soothed Denise during her worst days and provided the emotional support that had kept her going through the hardest times. Now, near the end of the year, Denise had changed enough so that even her mother had trouble understanding what was making her tick.

Rather than being unusual or an exception, this estrangement from family and friends Denise experienced is typical of interns in the latter half of their year. "My family doesn't understand what I'm going through," they tell each other (because no one else would understand). "I can't talk to them anymore." And so, they don't talk to them; they don't talk to anyone ... except fellow interns. To some extent, both Hal and Scott expressed some of these feelings in their diaries, and nearly every intern I've ever spoken with has felt it.

Unfortunately, it is not until after their training has ended that house officers come to recognize what's happened to them during their internship. But by then, it's too late. At least some of the damage that results from the estrangement and isolation becomes permanent and irreparable. These changes are the reason that some physicians seem uncaring and unfeeling to their patients later in their careers.

At the end of my vacation in April 1980, I returned to Boston rested, relaxed, and as ready to go as I could possibly have been. Most important, I had hope; it appeared as if I might sail smoothly until the academic year came to its end. But the sense of smooth sailing is at best an illusion to house officers. No matter where they're working, no matter through what service they're rotating, disaster lurks around every corner. When working with hospitalized patients, there's always the chance that one of the patients is going to get very sick very fast. When that happens, the life of the intern, as well as the lives of your patient and her family, can instantly turn to turmoil.

11

M A Y

The Eleventh Rotation:
Critical Caring

Much of the day-to-day aggravation that occurs in the lives of interns results from those frustrating hours spent coping with attending physicians, nurses, lab technicians, and the rest of the hospital staff. But aggravation is only a minor annoyance to the house officer, an annoyance that's not too different from that experienced by people in other professions. No, the run-of-the-mill aggravation caused by these contacts would easily be tolerable if it weren't for those moments of sheer terror that really cause interns and residents to develop serious ulcers. For the intern working in an intensive care unit, emergency room, or similar setting, acute medical crises wait around every corner.

The first time I realized how stressful the life of an intern can be occurred when, as a thirteen-year-old, I read Dr. X's *Intern*. In the part of his diary kept during one of his rotations through surgery, Dr. X describes assisting an attending surgeon operating on a patient with a large abdominal mass. During the operation, the surgeon's scalpel accidentally nicked the abdominal aorta, the main blood vessel carrying blood from the heart to the lower half of the body. In vivid detail, Dr. X describes how a gush of blood spurted out of the abdominal cavity, splashing upward onto the fluorescent lights that illuminated the surgical field. Within minutes, everything, the surgeons' gloves, gowns, faces, the surgical drapes and lights, were covered with a layer of the patient's blood. Panicking, the surgeon and intern attempted to stop the flow of blood from the aorta, but everything they tried failed. The bleeding continued and, within minutes, the patient exsanguinated and died.

That image of the intern and the attending surgeon standing together, helplessly, as the patient bled out, so well represented in the words of Dr. X, has stayed with me ever since. And although many things have changed in the lives of interns since Dr. X began his training over thirty years ago, these emergency situations continue to cause the most stress.

The emergency room is the place where most life-and-death dramas begin. The frightening thing about working in an emergency room is that, at any moment, with little or no warning, virtually anything can come walking or rolling through the front door. And no matter what the disaster, be it an airplane crash, factory explosion, or apartment house fire, the emergency room is the triage site, the initial port of entry leading to the intensive care units and operating rooms of the hospital. As a doctor working in an emergency room, it's necessary to stay alert and be ready for action.

Occasionally, some of the crises that start in the ER spill over into the rest of the hospital and actually prove harmful to the health of the house officer. Such a situation occurred to Gordon

Ellman, one of my medical school classmates who went on to do a residency in surgery at the hospitals affiliated with the Schweitzer School of Medicine.

During November of his internship year, Gordon was assigned to the surgery service at the Bronx Episcopal Medical Center, a rundown hospital in one of the worst sections of the south Bronx. At that time, in the area around the hospital, a turf battle raged between two rival street gangs, one composed of African-Americans, the other Puerto Rican. While on call one night, Gordon and the resident covering him were paged to the emergency room stat. When they arrived, they found the ER staff working on a young Puerto Rican man stabbed in his chest and abdomen at least a hundred times.

"It was right out of *West Side Story*," Gordon told me during one of our occasional phone conversations that year. "You know, the Jets and the Sharks were having a rumble, and this unfortunate citizen got the worst of it. By the time his pals managed to get him to the hospital, he was already pretty much dead. He'd nearly bled out, he was pale and blue and barely breathing, he had a thready pulse and a blood pressure of nothing over less than zero. He was in shock, and on top of all that, it looked like he had a tension pneumothorax. Plus, we had no idea what was going on in his belly: We stuck a needle in there and got bright red blood out, so for all we knew, every one of his internal organs was lacerated and bleeding like crazy. He was a mess. I was pretty sure he'd bought the farm, but my resident thought we had a chance of saving him, so he came up with a plan: First, we'd put a chest tube into him to reexpand his lung and pump a shitload of blood into him to get his blood pressure up into a range that's consistent with human life; then, we'd take him to the OR and explore his belly, and hope we could control the bleeding. Pretty straightforward, right?"

I agreed that it sounded pretty straightforward.

"So, anyway, we started in doing what needed to be done. By the time we had gotten down there, the ER docs had managed to get a big line into him [that is, an intravenous line with a large-bore needle], and the blood bank had already released six units of packed red cells, so they began pouring in the blood. My resident and I worked on the chest tube. We pushed the sucker in, got hit with a blast of air, and the guy's color immediately got better. It was around that point that we started to stupidly believe this guy had something like a chance."

"Why stupidly?" I asked.

"Because of what happened later," Gordon answered. "After the ER docs got the six units of blood into him, the guy's blood pressure came up and pretty soon, it looked like he was stable enough to get him upstairs for the exploration. My resident called the OR, told them we were on our way, and with one of the ER nurses and a couple of med students, we began pushing the stretcher and all the equipment that was needed to keep the guy going out the back door of the emergency room toward the elevator.

"After we got him to the OR, I prepped the abdomen while my resident and one of the med students scrubbed. After the guy was ready, the resident came in and opened the belly. The whole thing was a mess; the belly was full of blood—they had sliced his innards to ribbons. We could see immediately that this was going to take the rest of the night. The resident told the anesthesiologist to call the blood bank and tell them to keep shipping up blood. He figured this was at least a forty- to fifty-unit procedure.

"Anyway, we settled in to work. With the med student sucking out the blood as fast as he could, the resident and I found the bleeders and tied them off. But blood was coming from everywhere, so it seemed like a complete waste of time to me. I guess we were making some headway, though, because eventually, the rate that the belly was filling up with fresh blood seemed to be slowing down a little.

"Things were moving along like that, we were all concentrating on the work we were doing when suddenly, I heard this ruckus coming from outside the OR. Now remember, this is about 2:30 in the morning, and we're the only OR in the suite that's in use. At that hour, there shouldn't be anyone else around there.

"In any case, I heard the noise and looked up just in time to see a whole shitload of guys come pouring through the door. They were these big black guys, and they were carrying knives and guns and stuff. The leader said, 'That's Sanchez, right?'

"I have to tell you, Bob, I was so shocked to see those guys in the OR, I couldn't figure out right away what was going on. I guess the medical student and the anesthesiologist were in the same boat as me, because we all just stared at them like they were crazy. But my resident understood; later on, he told me that this had happened to him once before, when he'd done his intern rotation at the BEPI [internese for Bronx Episcopal Medical Center]. Without hesitating, he looked up from the abdomen and told the guy, 'No, this isn't Sanchez. This is an eighty-year-old guy from a nursing home who ruptured his appendix. It's a fucking mess in here. Lots of blood and pus and stuff. Want to see?'

"The guy apparently didn't want to see. He yelled back, 'Then where the hell is Sanchez at?' The resident told him that Sanchez had died in the emergency room a couple hours before and, as far as he knew, his body was at that moment cooling off down in the morgue. The leader of the gang said that wasn't what he'd heard. The rumor was that the doctors had saved

Sanchez and brought him up to the operating room. 'Now we're here to finish him off,' the guy told us.

"My resident, cool as a cucumber, said, 'Well you heard wrong. Sanchez is down in the morgue. If you don't believe me, go down there and check it out yourself.' The guy tried to stare him down, but it was pointless. My resident was already back in the patient's belly, tying off more bleeders. When he finally yelled, 'Can I get some suction down here?' that finally broke our trances. The med student started sucking and I started tying off more bleeders. After a few seconds, the gang leader said, 'Let's go,' and they all disappeared out the door."

"Shit," I said. "They could have killed you. What'd you do then?"

"Well, the first thing that happened was, while my resident and this guy were discussing the situation, the circulating nurse slipped out of the OR and called security. You've never worked at the BEPI, have you?"

I told him I hadn't.

"Well, the place may be the world's worst shithole, but one thing they're good at down there is security. The BEPI has a spectacular security force. They have to: This kind of shit happens all the time. Anyway, the circulating nurse called security, they called in the city cops, and together, they got the black gang surrounded. Just to be on the safe side, the circulating nurse opened a second operating room and we moved our patient in there. We kept the original room set up as a decoy, to at least give us some warning if the guys came back."

"Did Sanchez make it through the surgery?" I asked.

"Sure did," Gordon told me. "You know the old saying, 'You can't kill shit.' We used up more than fifty units of blood, and we wound up working on him until 6:30 in the morning, but he came through it just fine. The sad thing is, it was probably all a waste. I'm sure the guy'll get his head blown off the minute he walks out of the hospital."

Crises in the emergency room were a part of the lives of the interns whose diaries made up *The Intern Blues*. In early November, Mark Greenberg recorded this entry, describing an event that occurred on his last day on call in the emergency room at Jonas Bronck Hospital during the October rotation:

I was on call in the pediatric emergency room last night and I learned an important lesson: If you want people to trust you and have faith in your judgment, it's probably not a good idea to come to work dressed like Bozo the Clown. I know, because I did come to work dressed like Bozo the Clown yesterday, and things didn't go all that well. In fact, it was one of the worst nights of my life.

I guess I should explain. Yesterday was Halloween. The day before, our on-call team talked it over and we all decided that, since we're pediatricians and Halloween is such a big holiday for kids, we should get into the spirit by coming to work dressed in costumes. To be honest, I thought it was a stupid idea from the very beginning, but since I'm only an intern, you can't expect me to tell my senior resident, "No, I think that's stupid, I think wearing a costume all day in the emergency room is a dumb idea."

So anyway, after I finished work on Friday night, I went home and tried to find my Bozo costume. I knew it had to be around somewhere. I'd had it since my first year of medical school. It was given to me by one of my classmates who'd found it buried in his closet during one of his housecleaning frenzies that he went through while he was studying for our neuroscience final. It consisted of an orange wig, a big glue-on nose that squeaked when you squeezed it, a big smock, and big clown shoes. There also was this makeup kit. My classmate was going to throw it out, but I figured, what the hell, maybe someday it would come in handy, so I took it and proceeded to lose it in my own closet.

After looking around for about a half hour, I finally found the thing, still in its original box, squashed into a corner of my closet. I took it out and put on the smock, shoes, and wig: They still looked good as new. Early Saturday morning, I got dressed in the costume, put on the makeup as well as I could, and looked in my mirror: I have to admit, I looked pretty stupid. But I guess that's the look I was trying to achieve, so I got in my car and came to the hospital.

I may have looked stupid, but when I reached the hospital, I found that compared to the other guys on call, I looked pretty conservative. Peter Carson, our senior resident who's about six feet three and weighs at least 250 pounds, was dressed as a ballerina, in a tutu, leotard, and size-thirteen toe shoes. I have no idea where he got any of this stuff. Terry Tanner, one of the junior residents, came dressed as the Pope; she spent the entire day blessing people and inviting them to kiss her ring. And two of my fellow interns came dressed as killer bees, wearing yellow and black body suits, long antennae, and these long stingers that looked like it was going to make sitting down kind of a challenge. Even Lucille Turner, the ER's crabby head nurse, made an effort, but frankly, her costume wasn't much of a stretch: She came dressed as the Wicked Witch of the West. All in all, we presented quite a picture to the sick and wounded of the Bronx.

Well, we looked like idiots, but at least the kids seemed to like it. They all looked kind of stunned when they first came in from the waiting room and saw us. But almost immediately, each of the kids began to smile, and pretty quickly, they started to laugh. We had bowls of candy spread around the place, and the kids were helping themselves (at least the ones who didn't come in with gastroenteritis). Most of the parents seemed skeptical: It's one thing to come to the emergency room after you've been kept awake all night by a screaming three-year-old to be seen by what you think is a competent, or at least a semicompetent, doctor. It's another, though, to have to go through all that and then wait an hour or two to finally be seen by Bozo the Clown. But I think, at least, most of the people left thinking that it was a good idea and weren't we a nice group of doctors to think of the kids.

The day was going on pretty well; I was even beginning to think that maybe this really was a good idea. That's when we got the phone call. It was about nine o'clock, right in the middle of the busiest time of the evening. We got a call from EMS saying that they were bringing in a traumatic arrest. So Bozo the Clown, the six-foot-three-inch prima ballerina, the Wicked Witch of the West, the Pope, and one of the killer bees each left the patients we were working on and started to get ready back in the trauma area.

After about two minutes, there was this loud commotion and there they were. The emergency medical technicians were pushing a stretcher. One of the techs was on the side, doing chest compressions, while the other was at the back of the stretcher, working the ambu-bag. With them hovering over the patient, it was hard to see at first who the patient actually was.

It turned out to be an eight-year-old boy. He'd been out trick-or-treating and, after stepping out into the street between two parked cars, he'd been nailed by a passing van. The driver of the van panicked and, not knowing what to do, slammed the thing into reverse. That caused the kid to be run over a second time.

Someone had called 911, and the ambulance had gotten there within ten minutes. They'd started CPR out on the street, but you could tell it wasn't doing the kid much good. He was pulseless and *apneic, and when they hooked him up to a monitor, he was flatline. He was clearly DOA.*

We figured it was probably pointless, but we did everything we could anyway. Peter Carson intubated the kid, Terry Tanner started pumping on his chest, and Bruce Davidson (one of the killer bees) and I tried to get a line into him. I managed to get a good one into his right arm, and we started pushing bicarb and epi, but nothing helped.

At about that point, the trauma surgeons came in and said they wanted to crack the kid's chest. None of us believed it would help, but we figured we had to give this kid every possible chance to survive; besides, when three surgeons walk up to you with scalpels in their hands and say they'd like to crack a patient's chest, it's hard to say no.

It took no more than two minutes to get the chest open, and when it was, it became clear that the code was over: We found that the kid had a bronchopleural fistula. The impact of the van had caused the left main stem bronchus, the main windpipe to the left lung, to tear in half; the oxygen that we were forcing into the boy's windpipe through the endotracheal tube was ending up in the pleural space outside the lung, causing a tension pneumothorax that just kept getting worse.

After seeing that, I walked out of the trauma area to get some air and the boy's mother was standing there less than ten feet away. She was literally being held up by one of the emergency room nurses. She said, "Doctor, how is he? How is my son? Is he going to be okay?" I didn't see any way out; I was too upset to come up with a lie. So that's when I, dressed in my Bozo wig, my Bozo makeup, my Bozo shoes, and my Bozo smock, which was now soaked through with her son's blood, told that woman that her boy had died.

She went crazy. She started crying and fell down on the floor. I felt like a total idiot standing there dressed like that and there was nothing, absolutely nothing, I could do to change anything. After a minute, one of the hospital administrators came in and he, the nurse, and I managed to lift the mother up off the floor. The administrator then led the crying woman out of the ER.

I left the emergency room, too; I just couldn't see another patient just then, not looking the way I did. I took the stairs up to the operating room's locker room, which was deserted. I went to the sink and scrubbed the blood and the stupid clown makeup off my face. I then took off the costume and put on a fresh set of scrubs. Before leaving, I bundled up the wig, shoes, and smock, and threw the whole bloody mess into the garbage can. I don't think I'll ever get dressed up as a clown again. And next year, if I'm on call on Halloween again, I am not going to get dressed up.

Although the emergency room is a universal horror show, we pediatricians have our own private hell. It is in the delivery room where, at any hour of the day or night, we can be presented with a tiny, critically ill infant whose life is literally in our hands. Unquestionably, during their hours of sleep, the delivery room figures in more nightmares experienced by pediatric house officers than any other part of the hospital.

That was certainly true for me. As mentioned in the first chapter of this book, I spent the first month of my internship in a neonatal intensive care unit. By the end of that month, I had developed this recurring nightmare, which followed me through the remainder of my training: I'm standing alone, the only pediatrician in the delivery room, waiting to be handed a baby delivered through thick meconium. I quickly place the baby on the room's warming table, dry off the mec-stained amniotic fluid that covers his body, and begin trying to intubate him. But I can't find the vocal cords, which serve as the landmark through which the breathing tube must be passed. Using the laryngoscope, I search and search, but I just can't find them. And as time passes, the baby, who is not breathing, becomes limp and lifeless, his heart rate dropping to zero, and, ultimately, he dies.

I haven't had it in years, but I still feel queasy just thinking about this dream. And though this scenario never actually happened to me, it came pretty damned close to coming true on one occasion. It was during my second year of residency. I was working in the well-baby nursery at Schweitzer's University Hospital. As in the dream, I got called to the delivery room to attend the birth of a baby because of thick meconium. About an hour before, this woman's membranes had ruptured, and a stream of meconium-stained amniotic fluid had emerged. The fetus, who'd been closely monitored since that time, had shown no signs of distress, and although nothing horrible was suspected, the obstetrician wanted a pediatrician in the room to assure that the airway was clear.

Arriving in the DR a few minutes before the baby emerged, I introduced myself to the parents and explained what I was doing there. They told me this was their first baby and they were very excited about the event. The father had a camera with him and was planning to take pictures of the entire event. I told him I'd do my best to smile when he told me to.

When the delivery seemed imminent, I picked up a warmed receiving blanket and took my place beside the obstetrician, an attending physician who'd been working in the hospital forever. I knew there was a problem when I heard him say, "Uh-oh." But without another word, he finished the delivery, tied off and cut the umbilical cord, and handed the baby over to me. "What's that going on in her belly?" he asked me, under his breath.

I knew immediately what it was: The baby had a huge omphalocele, a defect in the wall of the abdomen. Because of the defect, most of this infant's abdominal contents, including her intestines, were situated in this sac outside of her body. I knew immediately that this baby was in trouble, that she was going to need surgery within the next few hours, and that I needed some backup. Unfortunately, that's when I froze.

This had never happened to me before, and it's never happened since. Something about that baby, about that huge defect in her abdomen, made me panic. I simply forgot what I was supposed to do. Standing there with the baby wrapped in the warm blanket cradled in my arms, I just stared off into space, as if in the midst of a seizure. After a few seconds, the obstetrician broke the spell. "Doctor, is anything wrong?" he asked. "Don't you want to get to work on this baby?"

I nodded at him, walked over to the warming table, plopped the baby down, and started to towel her off. But I couldn't remember what it was I was supposed to do next; I stood there looking at that huge defect in her abdomen, thinking about how it had happened and what additional problems might be associated with it. In the meantime, the infant had already aspirated a good deal of the meconium that had been lying in her mouth and nose and, by that point, was already experiencing some respiratory distress.

I'm convinced that had backup not arrived in the delivery room so quickly, that baby would have died with me standing by, helplessly staring at her. Luckily, all this happened in the middle of the afternoon, and as soon as the omphalocele had been seen, one of the delivery room nurses called the NICU to get the attending neonatologist to the DR stat. The attending arrived within two minutes. After pushing me aside, he assessed the situation and did everything that needed to be done. I continued to stand there, completely worthless and hopeless.

The baby was stabilized and brought to the NICU. She was extremely sick for the next two days, but eventually her breathing improved and, on the third day, she was taken to the operating room to repair her omphalocele. She spent that whole month and part of the next in the hospital, but eventually went home in good condition. No one said anything to me about my performance in the delivery room, but I knew I had screwed up big-time. Although I never saw that baby again and don't know what ultimately became of her, I've carried this terrifying memory with me ever since.

Life was no different for the three interns I followed in 1994 and 1995. Crises in the delivery room continue to occur with regularity, and no amount of regulation or restriction of work hours will ever change that. From his diary entry of December 29, here's Scott Lindsay's account of a night on call in the neonatal intensive care unit at West Bronx Hospital:

I was on call last night with Eric, the resident from my rotation on Infants' [the infants' unit at Mt. Scopus]. *The night was so slow, we finished the scut, went and got our own dinner—which is a real rare event when you're in the NICU—and watched some TV in the doctors' lounge. Unfortunately, the TV doesn't have an antenna, so the only station we can get is a Spanish station that broadcasts from New Jersey. Eric figured it was better than just sitting and watching fruit flies mating on the rotting bananas somebody left sitting on the windowsill, so we watched the local New Jersey news in Spanish, and Eric and I had a long talk. It was a great evening.*

We went to bed at around midnight. We'd done everything that needed to be done and everyone was stable, including the nurses.

my progress notes. Honestly, the night went so fast, I didn't even realize how much time was passing. . . .

Though stressful, these critical-care situations account for less than 10 percent of the time interns work in the hospital. And by the end of May, everything, even these gut-wrenching incidents, seems a little more tolerable. Because after May comes June, and as every house officer who reaches June says, "They can't hurt me now!"

12
J U N E

The Last Rotation:
The Wheel Begins to Turn

Getting up to go, feeling sad and happy both at once, I asked him:
"Hey, ace intern, notice anything different about me?"
He looked me up and down and then said, "Damn, Basch! NO
BEEPER!"
"They can't hurt me now."
"There it is, man."
"There it is."
I walked out of the on-call room, down the corridor, down the
stairs.

Dr. Roy Basch, ex-intern,
leaving the House of God for the last time

Part 1: The End of the Beginning

On July 1, the evolutionary wheel of residency training completes its rotation; the senior residents become attendings, the
junior residents become seniors, and the interns leave behind
their positions at the bottom of this pathologic food chain and

assume the supervisory position of junior residents. But although the cycle is completed in July, the anxiety caused by these changes is most strongly felt in June.

Senior residents depart from the shelter of the ivory tower and enter the unforgiving world of managed care, where concerns about salary, overhead, malpractice coverage, and regular office hours replace those about making it through long nights intact. At least, these are some of the concerns that occupy those lucky enough to leave their residencies with an actual job.

That's right. Although it may seem unbelievable and improbable, because of shifts caused by managed care's emphasis on primary care, over the past few years more and more residents who spent years training in medical and surgical subspecialties have found themselves unemployed and unemployable after the completion of their educations. One of the most striking and depressing examples of this unfortunate trend occurred this past July to Larry and Andrea Stark, a couple who attended the Albert Schweitzer School of Medicine in the late 1980s.

After graduating from Schweitzer, Larry and Andrea, who met during their first year of medical school and married during their third, went off to do separate residencies. Andrea, who chose a career in pediatrics, remained with our program in the Bronx, while Larry went to Columbia Presbyterian Medical Center in Manhattan, where he began the long, arduous training required to become an otolaryngologist. After she'd finished her three years of training, Andrea stayed on at Schweitzer, getting a job in our clinic and working as an attending pediatrician. But near the end of the fourth of his five years of ENT training, Larry became disenchanted with his chosen field. "It's the same thing every day," he told me once during that period. "Wax in the ears, hearing loss, tumors, over and over again. There's no diversity, nothing exciting ever happens. You're never called on to do anything creative." Around this time, Larry decided that what he really wanted to do was become a plastic surgeon. So early in the fifth and final year of his ENT residency, he filled out applications for training programs in plastic surgery.

I remember thinking how insane Larry must have been. I couldn't then, and I can't now, imagine how anyone who's finished one residency could possibly consider doing a second one. Personally, I was so beat up after finishing my training that, following my last night on call as a senior resident, I vowed that I'd never enter an on-call room again for the rest of my life. But Larry Stark was motivated; he didn't care about the sacrifices he and his family would have to make; he wasn't concerned about starting over and having to spend the next four years working his ass off during nights and weekends while collecting low pay. He simply didn't want to spend his life as a practicing otolaryngologist. He wanted to be a plastic surgeon.

By the time he applied, positions in plastic surgery residencies had become scarce and, therefore, highly competitive. After applying to more than fifty programs, Larry was accepted by only one. With no choice, the couple moved their family, which now included two young sons, to Syracuse, New York. Larry began his second residency, while Andrea, who had no trouble finding a job as a pediatrician, began work in a clinic.

Finding that he enjoyed plastic surgery a great deal more than he had ENT, Larry decided that, following completion of his training, he would try to get a job in academic medicine. He liked the atmosphere of teaching hospitals. He enjoyed the challenge of teaching residents and medical students, of doing research. So in the summer of 1995, at the start of the last of his nine years of residency training, Larry sent letters advertising his availability and copies of his curriculum vitae to the big teaching hospitals throughout the Northeast.

Three months passed. He received no calls or letters expressing interest.

By late November, becoming a little concerned, Larry followed up his initial letters with phone calls. He was told by one department chairman after another that although on paper he looked incredibly well qualified, they were sorry, but they simply had no jobs available. A little more concerned, Larry widened his circle, mailing out letters and CVs to teaching hospitals throughout the United States.

Three more months passed. Again, he received no calls or letters.

By February, Larry decided that although academic medicine was still his first choice, he could certainly survive happily in private practice. Once again, he sent out letters and copies of his CV, this time to a large number of plastic surgeons in private practice throughout the United States.

Three more months passed. There seemed to be no interest at all.

In May, the couple began to panic. Anticipating they would be leaving Syracuse in June, Andrea had given notice to the head of the clinic at which she'd worked for the past four years. Although he told her how sorry he was to see her go and how difficult he believed she'd be to replace, the reality was that the clinic hired a new pediatrician to fill her spot the very next week. As they sat at their kitchen table in late May, staring at each other, they realized for the first time that in one short month, they both would be unemployed.

In June, his back now against the wall, Larry tried some desperate moves. He talked to the chairman of plastic surgery in Syracuse about remaining on for an additional year of training as a clinical fellow. The chairman told him that he'd love to have Larry's services, but since there was no salary line for such a position, he'd have to work for nothing. He called the chairman of ENT at Columbia, the man who had been his program's director during his first residency, and asked if any similar position was available. He was given the same response.

In July, their lease up, the Starks moved from their apartment in Syracuse to Andrea's parents' house in New Jersey. They are currently both out of work. Between them, they have a total of eight years of college, eight years of medical school, and twelve years of postgraduate medical training. Getting to this, they have accumulated more than $200,000 in education loans. They are currently collecting unemployment benefits.

I spoke with Andrea recently. She told me their current plan is to move to Savannah, Georgia, a city in which they believe the cost of living is relatively low. Andrea is actively searching for a job in a pediatric clinic; Larry is planning to start his own private practice in plastic surgery. In this age of managed care, Larry's plan is a risky endeavor. He figures, though, that he has little to lose, except another $100,000 or so, the estimated cost of starting a new medical practice from scratch.

Although in June, senior residents have to deal with facing the cold, cruel realities of life outside the insulated world of academic medicine, the interns have real concerns about their future, as well. Moving from well-trained scut-dogs to supervisors of inexperienced scut-dogs can be a frightening transition.

In June, as the days of their first year of training wind down, virtually every intern has the same fear: I've spent the last year doing nothing but running scut. Since I haven't learned anything, since I haven't even opened a book or read a journal article since the day I graduated from medical school, how can I possibly be expected to teach new interns what they need to do?

Like so many other things about internship, there's been lit-tle change in this attitude since *The Intern Blues*. No Bell Commission regulations have made soon-to-be second-year res-idents feel less inadequate. Here's an excerpt from Andy Baron's diary from *The Intern Blues*, dated June 24, 1986:

> *Internship is supposed to be an important educational experience, but I'm still not sure what I've learned ... I definitely don't feel ready to be a second-year resident yet. I don't feel ready for that next step, that sudden acquisition of great responsibility where I'm the one who has to make the decisions and oversee the interns. I've gotten pretty good at doing what I've been called on to do as an intern. I have my own opinion now about how things should be done, but I don't argue much if I disagree with the residents or the attendings. They've got their jobs to do and I've got mine.*

And flashing ahead nine years, here's a portion of Scott Lindsay's diary entry dated June 18, 1995:

> *My second-year residency is rapidly approaching, and I have to admit, my overall knowledge is not quite what I wanted it to be at this point in my training. I'm going to be a resident soon; I'm going to have power over interns, and I'll be the one who's expected to teach them and lead the team. I'm definitely going to have to do a lot more reading in my second year; since starting last July, I've barely even opened a book. I feel comfortable right now with what I have to do as an intern, but being a resident? It's a lot of responsibilities.*
>
> *It'll be good in one sense. With these new responsibilities comes the loss of a lot of the dirty work: less scut, no more progress note writing, no more renewing orders. That's all great! Plus, as a resi-*

dent, you get more respect from the nurses (although there are so many nurses who aren't talking to me anymore, I may have to change my name).

But these interns' assessment of their abilities is way off base. Although it may be true that they never had time to open a textbook or read a journal, the amount of information they've picked up during the course of their twelve rotations is phenomenal. During this relatively brief period, they've been transformed from outsiders into physicians. They've developed skills that allow them to manage both the patient and his or her disease; they've learned how to interpret impressive amounts of data and precisely how to react to them. Perhaps most important, they've learned how to think on their feet—they've gained the ability to respond to any crisis at any hour of the day or night.

And of course, because they've learned all this, every one of the interns I've followed through the years, even those who were absolutely convinced they couldn't possibly have learned enough to supervise new interns, became a good resident. It's not until the moment the new interns show up to start the first day of their first rotation that the old interns finally get some sense of how far they've come. As an example, here's an excerpt from Mark Greenberg's last diary entry, following his last night on call in the NICU at West Bronx Hospital, dated June 28, 1986:

This morning at about eight o'clock, I was . . . walking around the unit whistling and jabbing great big needles into my wonderful patients, because I love them all so much [actually, Mark was doing his routine morning blood-drawing rounds], *and this guy who looked lost and scared to death came in and asked, "Is this the nursery?" Guess who he was. He was . . . an intern. He was* the new intern who was scheduled to be on call in the NICU today! And I didn't know who the fuck he was! Because he's brand-new!

I told him he was in the right place, and I showed him where to get a set of scrubs and then I showed him the patients. Ha ha. What fun that was! Of course, while I was doing this, I made sure to stay between him and the door at all times, because I was positive that at some point or other he was going to bolt, leave the hospital, and never come back, and I'd have to stay and be on call again. But he didn't leave. He was really nervous, but he seemed very enthusiastic. It was like I was talking to a member of a completely different species on the evolutionary tree. He took notes on this clean pad on this brand-new clipboard. He didn't ask me any questions, and I'm convinced he didn't understand a single word I said to him.

Is it possible that I was really like this poor guy a year ago? It seems hard to believe.

Part 2: "They Can't Hurt Me Now!"

Suddenly, it's over. One morning, the sun rises, the last night on call comes to its end, and the academic year is finished. The young doctor who entered the ward to take call the night before as an intern leaves as a junior resident.

What an anticlimax that morning is. The end of my internship was one of the biggest letdowns I've ever had. I'd looked forward to that day for so long, had dreamed about it during the nights I'd managed to get to sleep, had counted first the weeks, then the days, then finally the hours until I'd awaken from this nightmare. And then the day arrived; I finished my work, signed out to the new intern who had the bad luck of being on call the very first day of his internship, returned my beeper to the medical center's communication office, and, by 3:30 P.M., I was officially done.

On the afternoon of that last day, the pediatric department was sponsoring a party for those of us fortunate enough to be finishing, as well as those unfortunate enough to be starting. Set up in the hospital cafeteria, it had everything anyone could possibly want: There was plenty of food, lots of loud music, a dance floor, and even champagne. Nearly the entire housestaff and most of the faculty turned out. It was quite a festive affair.

But I felt ambivalent about attending. On the one hand, after those twelve long months, the hospital's cafeteria was about the last place on Earth I wanted to be just then; on the other hand, I was one of the honored guests, and this was going to be the last time I'd ever have a chance to see a fair number of these people. I debated all this in my head and, at the last minute, decided to go.

I tried to have a good time, but I just couldn't bring myself to enjoy it. After about fifteen minutes, I'd had more than enough.

I said good-bye to my fellow interns. Some I knew I planned to keep in touch with; others I hoped never to see again. We'd been through a lot together, most of it really bad, and I knew I wouldn't miss them at all.

And so, at a little after 4:00 that afternoon, I walked out through the main entrance of the Boston Medical Center for the very last time (I vowed never to go through those doors again, and to this day, I've been successful in keeping that vow). Once out the door, I took a deep, cleansing breath—the first taste of freedom I'd had since the electric doors of St. Ann's Hospital had closed behind me now nearly a year before—and immediately headed for a place called the Recovery Room, a dark, cool bar located a couple of blocks away from the hospital, a seedy staff hangout I'd found myself in a few times during the year when I really needed to get away.

As I sat at the bar and sipped a beer, I felt an array of emotions. I was, of course, overjoyed, ecstatic that I'd finished this very difficult year. But deep inside, there was also an enormous feeling of emptiness; I had put so much into this internship, so many hours, so many sleepless nights and miserable days, so much energy, so much emotion, and now all of that was behind me. I had nothing to show for any of this, nothing except a series of nightmarish memories and a piece of parchment attesting that I had completed an internship in pediatrics at the Boston Medical Center.

I didn't have a great deal of time to sit in the Recovery Room and lick my wounds. I was tired, the result of having been on call the night before, and I had to get ready for our move back to the Bronx, where I'd be starting my residency in just a few days. By five o'clock, I was on the bus back to Watertown.

That solitary beer at the Recovery Room was my transitional event, the borderland between my life as an intern and life after internship. For Roy Basch, after he'd turned in his beeper and walked through the main entrance of the House of God for the last time, this is how he chose to separate himself:

> Finally free, and more free for having glimpsed the fear
> and jealousy of those trapped inside, I left the House of
> God for the last time. Feeling the warm sun on my face, I
> felt a weight in my hand: my black bag. What should I
> do with it? Give it to the nearest six-year-old kid and

start him on his way to the top? Give it to an underprivileged? No. I knew what to do. Like a discus, round and round and round it went, gathering momentum, until with a scream of bitterness and joy I launched it up and up into the hot fresh summer breeze and watched the glittering chrome instruments fall out in a rainbow and smash on the pavement below.

Like me, Mark Greenberg celebrated the end of his internship in a bar. From his last diary entry from *The Intern Blues*:

I finished rounding . . . at about ten and then we all gathered in the West Bronx library and the party started. A bunch of us were sitting in there, drinking champagne and getting soused. At ten in the morning! We stayed there until about eleven, when the bar across the street opened, and then we all went over there for brunch. It might seem strange that ten or twelve interns would be sitting around a bar drinking at eleven in the morning, but hell, we weren't alone. The place was packed! It wasn't only pediatrics that changed over today; medicine and surgery changed also, and everyone was in there, getting loaded. Anyway, we stayed until about two. I just came home to take a nap and get ready for the real partying, which will start tonight.

I thought when it was all over, I'd have all these great, profound thoughts about internship. I've been trying to think of something profound to say all day, but I can't come up with a single thing. Internship sucks, that's all there is to it. It just flat-out sucks. But hey, it's not my problem anymore. I'm no longer part of that lower class of humanity. I'm pretty sure that if you come to me in five years and ask me if I thought my internship was a good or a bad experience, I'll probably tell you it was bad, but there were a lot of good things about it. That's what happens to people when they stop being so depraved. Right now, I can assure you there is absolutely nothing good about internship. Nothing.

Nearly ten years later, Scott Lindsay's internship ended somewhat less dramatically. Here's his final diary entry, dated June 30, 1995:

My last day of internship. It's kind of anticlimactic. I'm so drained and tired, I don't even feel like celebrating. And I don't even have time to celebrate: Starting tomorrow, I'll be working in the emergency room at West Bronx for a few weeks. Just in time for firecracker season; I can't wait. Internship was interesting. I don't think I'd ever want to do anything like this ever again, but it definitely was an interesting learning experience. I don't really have much more to say.

Terminal sign off.

Epilogue

And so, on July 1, 1995, Denise, Hal, and Scott were magically transformed into residents. Like the interns I followed in *The Intern Blues,* Roy Basch in *The House of God,* and Dr. X from *Intern,* like every other medical school graduate who's participated in the exercise, they were permanently changed by the experience.

But every person who lives through an internship is changed in different ways. Denise Powers, who started out bubbly, energetic, and outgoing, ended the year staid and reserved. Having started out using his sense of humor and sarcasm as an early defense mechanism, Scott Lindsay, somewhere along the line, lost these important tools and ended the year more serious. And Hal Burkins, who, lacking Scott's important defense system from early on, began his internship as a trusting, caring, optimistic young doctor, became transformed into a frightened pessimist, unable to trust those around him. During the year, all three of these interns lost some important attributes: They lost confidence in themselves, their ability to interact lovingly with others, and their youthful sense of trust.

Internship will do this to you; it permanently changes you. Unlike other experiences in life, the effects of spending twelve months as an intern do not wear off in one, five, or apparently even twenty years. There were things I lost during my internship, as well, characteristics such as my idealism—a feeling that I was doing something important, using my skills to help my fellow man. This seemed to disappear during my on-call nights. Some people have told me that the loss of this feature was not the result of my training, but rather the natural effect of maturation, a consequence of growing up. I disagree; I'm different not just because I'm older, but because of what happened to me in Boston.

I'm not alone. As a result of their participation in the process designed to turn them into technically competent physicians, interns and residents are forced to surrender the very ideals that brought them to medicine in the first place. We come to medicine with little knowledge or skill, but filled with humanism and commitment. As we train and are transformed into intellectually capable physicians, we become jaded, bitter, and angry—angry at the hospital for demanding that we work so hard and so long, angry at the nurses and the rest of the staff who we believe treat us poorly, and, worst of all, angry at the patients, the very people whom we've come to medicine to help, whom we now view as our enemies, the force that has come between us and our ability to get to sleep.

In most cases, following the completion of their training, residents regain at least some of the positive attributes they had at the beginning of their medical school experience. But many physicians never recover their idealism. These doctors spend the remainder of their careers caring little about anything other than their income and their lifestyle.

The process is so destructive that even the positive defense mechanisms some interns come to employ to keep afloat during difficult times get sacrificed to the training process. A good example of this is an encounter that occurred in 1988 between myself and the resident whose internship diary formed the basis of the character Mark Greenberg in *The Intern Blues*.

It had taken me more than a year to transcribe and edit the

cassette-tape diaries of the three interns that formed the basis of that book. As I completed my work (and as the book's deadline rapidly approached), I sent each of the residents a copy of their transcripts. A few days later, I got an angry call from Mark. "You can't publish this crap," he yelled at me over the phone. "I never said any of this stuff."

"What stuff are you talking about?" I asked, a little surprised by his reaction.

"All this stuff," he continued yelling. "Almost everything you have coming out of my mouth. Like here, during February, when I was in the NICU. You wrote 'And then we walked around and he showed us these so-called patients. My God, those things weren't patients; they couldn't have been human; they weren't anything more than small packets of pus and protoplasm! These things would have to quadruple their weight in order to be classified as patients. Right now, they're nothing more than tiny portions of buzzard food.' Bob, I never would have referred to premies as 'small packets of pus and protoplasm' or 'tiny portions of buzzard food'!"

"You don't remember saying those things?"

"I never said them," he replied. "How could I remember saying them if I never said them?"

"You don't remember your internship very well, do you Mark?"

"I remember it fine," he replied. "I agree that things were rough for most of the year. But no matter how bad things got, I always showed respect for my patients. I'm sure of that."

"Mark, I hate to burst your bubble, but not only did you say those things, but I've got them on tape. Would you like me to play them back to you?"

"You can't have them on tape, because I never said them," he reiterated. "If you have someone saying this stuff on tape, then it must have been one of the other interns who said it."

We argued on like that for a while. Finally, I agreed to let Mark "fix" at least some of what he believed was wrong with his portion of the book. I used his edited transcript to revise the final manuscript. Unfortunately, the revised edition cut out some of the best and funniest sections of Mark's cynical view of his world. To me it was amazing that, after the passage of less than eighteen months, this man had completely suppressed what had happened to him during his internship.

Unfortunately, that's one of the main problems with trying to bring about a change of the residency training system: People who have lived through an internship can't remember what the experience was really like. While appearing on a talk radio program after *The Intern Blues* was published, I received a call from a surgeon who had finished his training during the early sixties. He was not happy that I was disparaging the institution of internship, a system that had successfully trained doctors for so many years and one that, at least in his opinion, had served him well. "My internship taught me how to think on my feet," he explained. "Because I was forced to work at all hours of the day and night, I can now be awakened at four in the morning and be able to function well and perform surgery if I have to." I mentioned to him that functioning well and performing surgery at four in the morning after you've been asleep for five or six hours is very different from being called on to do those things after you've been awake and working hard for nearly twenty-four hours. He didn't seem to see the difference.

The problem is not so much that physicians are forced to lose the humanity with which they come to medicine (although the impact of this should not be underestimated), but rather that the care they are able to deliver to patients at two, three, or four in the morning, when they've been awake and working consecutively for twenty, twenty-one, or twenty-two hours, cannot possibly be as skilled and well reasoned as it would have been twelve hours earlier. This was the conclusion reached by Sidney Zion.

But has any significant change occurred as a result of the Bell Commission regulations? Has limiting the number of hours house officers are allowed to work resulted in more doctors who have successfully maintained their humanity and idealism through the rigors of internship? Has it brought better care to patients hospitalized in New York State? Unfortunately, from observations both in our and other residency training programs—and from comparing the experiences of Hal Burkins, Scott Lindsay, and Denise Powers to those of Andy Baron, Mark Greenberg, and Amy Horowitz—I have to conclude that the answer to these questions is no.

The lives of the interns who began their training after the enactment of the Bell Commission regulations are no better than those of interns who trained prior to 1989. Although they may be better rested, the result of being on call every fourth night instead of every third, house officers today are still overstressed and quickly become depressed. And even the greater amount of rest is of little value; as Scott Lindsay said to me, "The benefit of every-fourth-night on call versus every-third-night on call is actually pretty meaningless. I mean, is beating your head against the wall for fifteen minutes really that much better than beating your head against the wall for thirty minutes?"

If anything, the new regulations have resulted in a deterioration in the care that hospitalized patients receive. As already mentioned, the rules governing the number of consecutive hours house officers are allowed to work have made it necessary to sign patients out to care providers who have not admitted them. This system of signing in and signing out has resulted in a perpetual game of telephone, a constant telling and retelling of the patient's history, physical, and lab results. As is inevitable in a situation like this, details are bound to be lost, lab values wind up deleted and/or changed, and plans consistently fall through the cracks. The patient, who is often not even sure which of the people who come to see him every day is actually his doctor, winds up paying the price of this discontinuity by having to answer the same questions many times, repeat tests, and spend extra hours or even days in the hospital.

Although it's usually only a nuisance, this discontinuity can have tragic consequences. Late last year, a forty-three-year-old woman was admitted to a hospital in New York City for surgery. She had recently been diagnosed with a tumor in her colon, and, during an operation, the surgeon's plan was to biopsy the tumor and, if found malignant, resect it. In order to perform the appropriate preoperative evaluations, the woman was admitted two days prior to the scheduled surgery.

The intern who admitted the woman began the workup. He scheduled an MRI, some X ray tests, and sent off some blood work. The next morning, the first intern, having completed his twenty-four-hour shift, signed out to a second intern, whose job it was to follow up on some of the tests that the first doctor had ordered. That night, after she'd accumulated the results of all the tests the first intern had signed out to her, the second intern wrote a pre-op note in the woman's chart, detailing the results of these pre-op tests. Then, early the next morning, the woman was brought to the operating room for surgery.

After her abdomen was opened, the tumor was quickly identified and a small section of it was sent to the pathology lab for frozen section (in which a slice of tumor is quickly frozen and then examined under a microscope for evidence of cancer). Unfortunately, the frozen section revealed that the tumor was cancerous. During the rest of the operation, a large section of bowel and its surrounding connective tissue and lymph nodes were resected.

While examining the colon and the surrounding tissue, the surgeon had reason to feel optimistic. The cancer appeared well-circumscribed, the margins of the bowel were intact, and the surrounding tissue looked clean. The surgeon realized that these were good signs; this appeared to be an isolated tumor caught before it had a chance to metastasize. If this actually turned out to be the case, if the pathologist found no evidence of tumor cells in anything but the mass in the colon, the woman would have a good chance for a complete cure.

But following completion of the colon resection, the surgeon, in examining the rest of the woman's abdomen, made a discovery that destroyed his optimism: He found that the woman's uterus was enlarged. Believing this to be evidence that the cancer, in spite of its clean, well-circumscribed appearance, had spread beyond the bowel and invaded the womb, he removed that organ and sent it to pathology.

After the operation had been completed and the woman had been sent to the recovery room, the surgeon received a frantic call from the pathologist. "That colon cancer you did this morning," the pathologist said, "were you aware of the fact that she was pregnant?"

"What?" the surgeon asked. "What are you talking about?"

"The uterus you sent us contained a ten-week fetus."

"That's impossible," the surgeon replied. "I had my resident send off a pregnancy test when she was admitted. The test came back negative."

"You better check the test again," the pathologist said. "Somebody made a mistake."

In checking the hospital's computer, the surgeon discovered that a pregnancy test had been sent, but it had not been negative, as he had been led to believe. Rather, the test results had never been received by the house officer. Because of the game of telephone that occurred, the second intern had never even been told of the test. She never checked its results.

Seven years after the new regulations went into effect in New York State, it's clear to just about everyone involved that, although the Bell Commission's heart might have been in the right place, the system just doesn't work. What should be done?

First, the commissioner of the Department of Health in New York State must recognize that the regulations have failed and immediately convene a panel of experts to study the issue of residency reform. Individuals on this committee should include not just attending physicians and house officers, but representatives from all parts of the community that have direct interaction with house officers, including hospital administrators, nurses, members of the ancillary staff, and, most important, patients. The committee must study not only the issues raised in this book, but the larger issue of how managed care will impact both the way doctors are trained and the future of the delivery of health care in the state.

As their first act, the committee should scrap the Bell Commission's regulations and begin again. But in reconstituting residency training, what should they strive for?

First, there's the issue of hours. Although many have argued in the past that to be well trained, interns and residents need to work excessively long hours, the fact is that, with the exception of careers in surgery, there is absolutely no convincing evidence that this is true. There is no reason that schedules that allow house officers to work fifty or sixty hours per week couldn't be designed, schedules that would prevent young doctors from having to work more than twelve hours during a single shift. This is currently the way the nursing schedule in many ICUs operate; there's no reason that the situation with residents could not emulate a system that works so well with nurses.

In reducing further the number of hours that house officers work, nonphysician professionals, such as nurse practitioners and physician's assistants, will play a larger role in providing care for hospitalized patients. To best utilize these nonphysician professionals, it might be wise to scrap the conventional method of providing coverage on a ward and develop a new system. Rather than having a resident supervising three or four interns who are responsible for all patients on a ward, as is now the case, why not pair interns with physician's assistants or nurse practitioners to create a dyad? These dyads, to be supervised by an attending physician, would be responsible for the total care of a small group of patients. By limiting the number of professionals responsible for the care of an individual patient, most of the oversight errors would be eliminated.

Cutting the hours that house officers work to this more reasonable number will go a long way toward improving the situation. But as was the case with the Bell Commission regulations, restricting hours alone is simply not enough. It must be recognized that the work done by interns and residents—the management of critically ill patients—is stressful and, in the long run, can be quite damaging. In addition to this, an attempt must be made to help house officers cope with the stress. As such, counseling opportunities must be made more available, and house officers should be encouraged to participate in these services.

These suggestions are just a start. It is clear that to train effective physicians for the future, the entire structure of residency training throughout the United States must undergo a revolution. But the first step on the road to that revolution is recognition that the old system no longer works. To underscore this, here's Hal Burkins's final diary entry, dated June 29, 1995:

I'm finishing my last post-call day as an intern. Last night went as most nights have gone: some sleep, some work, a lot of worrying. I can't say I'm either sad or sorry it's over!

Looking back over the year, I guess there were some great moments, but they were few and far between, and right now, I'm having trouble remembering most of them. There definitely were some good times, and they always involved patients, times when I knew my work made a real difference in people's lives. . . . But most of those memories have been washed away by the many bad times: the nights on call when I would have rather been anyplace else on Earth than in the hospital; those post-call days when I was dead tired, but still had to slug it out with idiotic nurses who were lazy and stupid and didn't have a clue what it was like to be standing in my shoes; and that period back during the winter when I got sick and just couldn't function.

The worst part of it, I think, was the fact that I became so separated from people: I knew nobody could understand what I was going through, not my parents, not my friends, sometimes not even my wife. Only other interns could understand, and since they were going through the same crap I was, they weren't going to be very helpful. There were some times during the year, especially during some of those long, long nights, when I felt more alone than I've ever felt before. It was very, very scary.

But I made it. I survived my internship, which I now understand is quite an accomplishment. I'm sure I wouldn't have made it had it not been for the support of my wife. Even though she didn't always understand what was happening to me, Robin was always there. She made it possible for me to make it through this year. I simply can't thank her enough for what she's done for me, being there for me, listening to me, making my lunches, doing the laundry, propping me up when I was down, taking care of me.

Looking back on the year, I guess I have to admit that internship has taken me from medical student to physician. I now think differently, I act differently, and I react differently than I did just twelve months ago. The question is, Was what I had to give up worth what I've gained? I don't know. I may never know.

Glossary

A

Abdominal aorta:
The portion of the aorta (the largest blood vessel in the body) that passes through the abdomen.

Acidosis:
A buildup of acid in the bloodstream. Acidosis can result from a number of pathologic conditions, most of them pretty serious.

Ambu-bag:
A device used to force air into the lungs; consists of a mask that covers the mouth and nose and a rubber bag that, when squeezed, generates a gust of air under pressure. Used in respiratory arrests.

Amyloidosis:
A rare disease of unknown etiology characterized by the accumulation of a protein known as amyloid in various organs. Over time, the amyloid interferes with the functioning of those organs, leading ultimately to death.

Anticoagulant:
A medication used to inhibit the clotting of blood. Used in patients with deep vein thrombosis in an attempt to prevent pieces of the thrombus (or clot) from breaking off and

travelling to the lungs, where they can cause a pulmonary embolus.

APCs:

Abbreviation for atrial premature contractions, a disturbance in the rhythm of the heart.

Apnea:

Failure to breathe. Interns sometimes say that death is the ultimate apneic episode.

Asthma room:

The area of the emergency room in which patients with asthma are treated.

Atropine:

A drug used for many purposes, including increasing the heart rate in patients with bradycardia (a slow heart rate).

Aveinic:

"Internese" (that is, part of the intern's private language) for "having no veins." Aveinic patients present a serious problem when they need to have blood drawn or IVs started.

B

Bagging:

Internese for the act of forcing air into the lungs of a patient having difficulty breathing. Patients are bagged using an ambu-bag (see above).

Bell Commission:

The committee, convened by New York State's Department of Health and headed by Dr. Bertrand Bell, that issued a series of regulations governing house-officer working conditions. After adoption by the New York State legislature, the Bell Commission regulations (also called the 405 regulations) went into effect on July 1, 1989.

BEPI:

Internese for the Bronx Episcopal Medical Center, a facility in the south Bronx.

Bicarbonate:

A drug used in patients with acidosis (see above).

Blood gas:

A test done on a sample of arterial blood that tells the amount of oxygen and carbon dioxide within the body.

"Bought the farm":

Terminal event. Other intern euphemisms for dying include "kicked," "boxed," and, my personal favorite, "went to Chicago."

BPD:

Internese for bronchopulmonary dysplasia, a disease of the lungs that predominantly affects premature babies who have spent time on a ventilator.

Bronchiolitis:

Disease of the lungs, usually caused by a virus, that causes respiratory distress. Resembling asthma in many ways, bronchiolitis only occurs in children under one year of age.

Bronchopleural fistula:

A leak in the main air tube that causes air to leak into the pleural cavity, which, in turn, causes a tension pneumothorax, and very often death.

C

Cardex:

A file kept by the nurses on which all pertinent information regarding the patient is kept. The doctor's orders are listed on the cardex, as well as loads of other important facts.

CBC:

Complete blood count. A blood test to examine the content of hemoglobin, red blood cells, and white blood cells within a sample of blood.

Cefuroxime:

A commonly used antibiotic.

Chest tube:

A surgical tube passed through the chest wall and into the pleural space in an attempt to expand a collapsed lung.

Committee of Interns and Residents:

The house officers' union.

Compazine:

An antiemetic drug (used to prevent vomiting).

Conjunctivitis:

Pinkeye. An inflammation of the conjunctiva of the eye.

Coronary artery aneurysm:

Condition in which the wall of one or more of the arteries that carry blood to the heart balloons out and weakens. Often a result of Kawasaki disease, coronary artery aneurysms can cause heart attacks and sudden death.

Coumadin:

An oral anticoagulant. Coumadin can cause birth defects and therefore is contraindicated during pregnancy.

Cracking the chest:

The surgical opening of the chest wall in order to gain access to the heart and lungs.

Crump:

To deteriorate rapidly.

Cytomegalovirus:

A virus that can infect the fetus, causing congenital malformations.

D

Deep vein thrombosis:

Inflammation of a vein, usually in the thigh, leading to the formation of a blood clot. Dangerous, because if not treated, portions of the clot can break off and travel through the bloodstream to the lung, where it can cause a pulmonary embolus.

Dexedrine:

Speed. Used by Dr. X to stay awake and functional during one particular weekend when he developed the flu.

di George syndrome:

A series of congenital malformations leading to immune deficiency, severe heart disease, disturbances of calcium metabolism, and unusual facial features.

DKA:

Diabetic ketoacidosis. A severe metabolic abnormality that occurs in diabetics who have a marked buildup of sugar in their blood. If not cared for correctly, may lead to death or brain damage.

DNR:

Do not resuscitate.

Doctor's orders:

Instructions to the nursing staff about the care of hospitalized patients. Doctor's orders are written upon admission of the patient to the ward and are abridged as the patient's medical condition evolves.

DRGs:

Abbreviation for diagnosis-related groups. Refers to the amount of reimbursement a hospital will receive from an insurance company for the treatment of a specific condition. Because this provides an incentive to discharge patients prematurely, DRGs have revolutionized the way hospitals operate.

Dump:

Internese for the inappropriate transfer of a very sick patient from one service to another. "Dumps" can only be countered by a "bounce back," in which a reason is found to transfer the patient back to his or her original service.

E

EKG:

Electrocardiogram. A test in which the electrical activity of the heart is examined.

Electrolytes:

Some blood chemicals; include sodium, potassium, bicarbonate, and chloride.

Endotracheal tube:

A tube passed through the larynx and into the main breathing tube that allows the individual to be placed on a respirator.

F

Fascinoma:

Internese for an interesting case.

G

Glycogen storage disease:

A genetic disorder in which sugar is stored in the liver and other organs.

GOMER:

A mnemonic for "Get Out of My Emergency Room." Used by house officers to describe senile patients.

GOMERE:

The feminine form of GOMER.

GORK:

A mnemonic for "God Only Really Knows." Usually used to describe a patient who has suffered significant brain damage.

H

Hemangioma:

A tangle of blood vessels that can be found anywhere in the body, but often is seen on the skin.

Heparin:

An anticoagulant. Unlike Coumadin, which causes birth defects, Heparin is safe for use during pregnancy. Unfortunately, because it's inactive when taken orally, heparin must be administered by injection.

Hepatosplenomegaly:

Enlargement of the liver and spleen.

Hickman line:

A surgically placed, indwelling IV line that can be used for weeks or months. Usually used in patients with cancer who are receiving chemotherapy.

Horrenderoma:

Internese for a horrible case.

Hydrocephalus:

Dilatation of the ventricles of the brain, which can lead to increased intracranial pressure.

Hypoxia:

A deficiency of oxygen in the blood. May lead to brain damage.

I

Immune globulin:

Medication injection in an attempt to prevent an infection from occurring. For instance, it's used in people who have been stuck with needles from HIV-infected patients in an attempt to kill off the virus before it has a chance to cause an infection.

Intracranial bleed:

A hemorrhage into the brain; often causes brain damage or death.

Intubate:

Procedure in which an endotracheal tube (see above) is inserted through the vocal cords and into the main breathing tube.

IUGR:

Intrauterine growth retardation. Failure to grow properly during fetal life.

J

Joubert syndrome:

A rare congenital malformation syndrome that causes severe mental retardation.

K

Kaposi's sarcoma:

A form of cancer that commonly occurs in individuals who have AIDS.

Kawasaki disease:

A condition of unknown etiology that affects young children and causes a host of symptoms and signs, including persistent high fever, swollen lymph nodes, redness of the mucous membranes of the mouth, a skin rash, and peeling of the skin around the fingertips. Patients with this condition can go on to develop coronary artery aneurysms (see above).

KUB:

A type of X ray in which the abdomen is examined (abbreviation for Kidneys, Ureters, Bladder).

L

Laminaria:

A spongelike substance that, when placed around the cervix, will cause it to spontaneously dilate. Used in elective abortions and, later in pregnancy, to induce labor.

Lasix:

A powerful diuretic medication. Because of its general usefulness in a whole host of conditions, it's sometimes called "Vitamin L" by house officers.

Late decels:

Late decelerations. A heart rate pattern that, when seen while performing fetal monitoring, implies that the fetus is in distress and needs to be delivered as an emergency.

Lithotomy:

The position in which a woman is placed in preparation for performing a pelvic exam.

LOL in NAD:

Internese (from Samuel Shem's *The House of God*) for "Little Old Lady in No Acute Distress."

LOS:

Internese (at least according to Scott Lindsay) for "Load of Shit."

Lymphadenopathy:

Enlargement of the lymph nodes.

'Lytes:

Internese for "electrolytes" (see above).

M

Main stem bronchus:

One of the two main tubes connecting the trachea and the lungs.

Managed care:

A system of healthcare provision that will undoubtedly destroy the medical care delivery system in the United States as we know it today.

Meconium:

The baby's first bowel movement; when meconium is passed while the baby is still in the womb, it is often a sign of fetal distress and can lead to respiratory problems if it is aspirated.

Meningitis:

Inflammation, usually caused by infection, of the lining of and the fluid that bathes the brain.

MRI:

Magnetic resonance imaging. An X ray–like test used to examine various internal structures.

N

Neurofibromatosis:

A genetically inherited disorder that can cause abnormalities of the skin, the central nervous system, and other organs.

NICU:

Abbreviation for neonatal intensive care unit.

NPO:

Abbreviation meaning nothing by mouth. Ordered for patients with intestinal abnormalities and patients who are pre-op (see below).

O

Omphalocele:

A congenital malformation in which the abdominal wall does not develop, and the abdominal contents protrude through the belly button.

OPD:

Abbreviation for outpatient department, composed of the ER and clinics.

Osteogenic sarcoma:

A cancer of the bone.

P

Pancytopenia:

Deficiency of all types of blood cells, both red and white.

PCP:

Pneumocystis carynii pneumonia. This type of pneumonia only occurs in individuals who are immunodeficient, with conditions such as AIDS.

PFC:

Abbreviation for persistence of fetal circulation, a complex physiologic abnormality encountered in sick newborns (i.e., those who have aspirated meconium).

PICU:

Pediatric intensive care unit.

Pneumothorax:

Collapse of a lung; must be treated by placement of a chest tube that drains out the accumulated air.

Polycystic kidney disease:

An inherited condition in which cysts form in the kidneys, causing them eventually to fail.

Premies:

Premature babies.

Proventil:

A drug used for the treatment of asthma; Proventil is frequently inhaled through a mist-producing device called a nebulizer.

Pulmonary embolus:

A blood clot that has travelled to the lung.

Q

QNS:

Abbreviation for quantity not sufficient.

R

RAD:

Abbreviation for reactive airway disease. Pretty much a synonym for asthma.

Respiratory syncytial virus:

A virus that causes, among other symptoms, bronchiolitis in young children. Also known as RSV for obvious reasons.

Ribovarin:

Medication used to treat RSV (see above).

S

SCID:

Abbreviation for severe combined immune deficiency, a rare, inherited condition. SCID can present in ways similar to AIDS, but is far less common.

Scrub suit:

Pajamalike outfit worn by surgeons in the operating room and house officers on call.

Scut:

A collective term for the routine work that an intern must do.

Sepsis:

Bacterial infection in the blood.

Sepsis workup:

A series of tests done when sepsis is being considered; includes blood, urine, and spinal fluid cultures.

SHPOS:

Internese mnemonic for subhuman piece of shit; a derogatory term used to describe some patients.

Stridor:

Noise heard on breathing in (inspiration), usually caused by narrowing of the trachea. Stridor is a symptom of croup, an illness caused by RSV (see above).

T

Teratogen:

A substance that can cause birth defects.

TPN:

Abbreviation for total parenteral nutrition, in which all the nutritional requirements are supplied via an intravenous route.

Transillumination:

Technique used to "light up" a particular structure. Used to diagnose pneumothoraces (see above).

Traumatic arrest:

Cessation of cardiac activity caused by a traumatic event (i.e., an automobile accident).

Turf:

Internese for sending a patient to another service. See "Dump," above.

U

UA:

(1) Abbreviation for urinalysis, a test performed on urine to see if a urinary tract infection is present; (2) abbreviation for umbilical artery, a blood vessel in the umbilical cord that carries blood from fetus back to mother.

V

Ventilator:
A machine that breathes for a patient.

Ventriculoperitoneal shunt:
Also known as a VP shunt. A plastic tube inserted into patients with hydrocephalus that drains excess spinal fluid from the ventricle of the brain to the peritoneal cavity of the abdomen.

W

Warfarin:
An anticoagulant; generic name for Coumadin (see above).

Index

abortion, 17–21
AIDS, 31, 111–30, 207
   effect on practice of medicine,
      111, 112, 113–14
   changes in attitude about, 129–30
   as "viral syndrome," 109, 113
Albert Einstein College of
   Medicine, xi, 147
Albert Schweitzer School of
   Medicine, xiii, xiv, 6, 53, 109,
   185, 232, 240
Anderson, Dr. Peter, xii, xiv
Andrews, Dr. Richard, 185, 187
asthma, 54–55, 87–88
attending physicians
   attitudes toward housestaff, 47,
      48–51
   goals of, 45

bacterial meningitis, 134–35, 138.
   See also Watson, Andre
Baron, Dr. Andy, xiii, xiv, 114, 129,
   178, 244
Bell, Dr. Bertrand, xi, xii, 147, 149,
   152, 156
Bell Commission, xi, xii, xiv,
   147–48, 149, 150, 154, 155, 156,
   255–60
   disregard for regulations of,
      154–55
   effect of regulations on quality of
      care, 155–56, 255–58

need for reform of regulations of,
   258
reaction to, 148–49
suggestions for reform of
   regulations of, 258–60
Berkowitz, Dr. Doug, 23–24
Boston Children's Hospital, 162,
   163
Boston Medical Center, 4, 35, 36,
   42, 44, 87, 95, 133, 160, 199, 200,
   247, 248
bronchiolitis, 114
bronchopleural fistula, 230
bronchopulmonary dysplasia, 56
Bronx Episcopal Medical Center,
   225, 226
Burkins, Dr. Hal, xiii, xiv, 2, 6, 61–62,
   63–64, 117–21, 130, 173–74,
   182–94, 202–4, 218, 251, 255
   and AIDS scare, 122–27
   attitude toward nurses, 188–89,
      190–91, 260
   depression of, 189–94
   effects of internship on, 251,
      260–61
   relationship with patients,
      28–33
   relationship with wife, 125, 127,
      128, 193, 201, 260, 261

café-au-lait spots, vii
Carson, Dr. Peter, 228, 230

Cintron, Dr. Erica, 54–55, 56, 58, 59, 218
conjunctivitis, 164
Cozza, Dr. Alan, 35–36, 37, 42, 44, 166, 168, 185

Davidson, Dr. Bruce, 230
deep-vein thrombosis, 168, 170
doctor-patient confidentiality, 30–31
Down syndrome, 95–96
"dumping" patients, 38, 42

Ellman, Dr. Gordon, 222–27
Erickson, Dr. Charles, 37, 39–41, 42
Evans, Art, 15–23
    approach to medical school of, 15–16
    first on-call experience of, 18–23

Firestone, Dr. Kathy, 191, 192
Flannagan, Dr. Mike, 160–61, 163

gangliosidosis, 107–8
The Girl Who Died Twice (Natalie Robins), 144
glycogen storage disease, 110
Goodman, Dr. Andrea, 10–15, 23
Greenberg, Dr. Mark, xiii, xiv, 1, 8–9, 114, 129, 205, 206–7, 227–31, 245–46, 252–54, 255
    coping mechanisms of, 178–80

Harris, Dr. Curt, 50–51. *See also* Reid, Dr. J. Cuthbert
Health and Hospitals Corporation, x–xi, xiv
hemangioma, 154
hepatitis, 31
hepatosplenomegaly, 109
Horowitz, Dr. Amy, xiii, xiv, 114, 129, 163–67, 170, 171–72, 173, 255
    coping mechanisms of, 178

hospital whites, 94
The House of God (Samuel Shem), 51–53, 89, 94, 104, 105–6, 107, 239, 248–49
hydrocephalus, 66–67

Intern (Dr. X), 105, 141, 158–59, 208–9, 221–22
The Intern Blues (Robert Marion, M.D.), xii, xiii, xiv, xv, 33, 113–14, 143, 178, 206, 215, 244, 254
interns
    attitude toward attending physicians, 51–53
    attitude toward nurse practitioners and physician's assistants, 55, 62–64
    attitude toward nurses, 75–76, 78, 80, 82–83, 188–89, 190–91, 216, 260
    attitude toward own illnesses, 79, 158–59, 159–60, 165
    average day of, 97–99
    coping mechanisms of, 14–15, 106–7, 122, 177–8, 180–81, 252–54
    decrease in number of, xiv
    depersonalization of patients by, 104–8
    deterioration of lifestyle and, 87–88, 92, 99–100, 176, 215–16, 260
    deterioration of relationships with others and, 103–4, 106–7, 108, 128, 177, 203–4, 216, 217, 218–19, 251, 260
    eating habits of, 87–88, 90–93, 97
    effect of AIDS on, 113–14, 116, 117, 122, 129–30
    effects of internship on, xii, 27, 217–18, 251–52, 254–55, 260–61
    fears of, xiii, 3, 198–99, 243–44

jargon of, 76, 105–6, 107–8, 113
pediatric, attitude toward eating,
    91–92
post-call experiences of, 98–99
pregnancy, attitude toward,
    168–70, 171–72
problems with attending doctors,
    43–44, 49–51, 53–60
problems with lab technicians,
    69–72
relationships with patients, 28–33
scut work and, 9–10, 45, 97, 98,
    137
stress and, 98, 222
surgical, attitude toward eating,
    90–91
internship, 143, 146–47, 245, 251–52
changes in, 93–95, 141, 207–8, 209
dress code, 94–95
effect of Bell Commission
    regulations on, 148–49, 155–56,
    255–58
effects of AIDS on, 112–14
history of concept, 142–43
Match Day and, 197–98
maternity leave and, 167–68, 172,
    173
intussusception, 61–62

Jefferson Hospital, 66
Johns Hopkins Hospital, origin of
    internship at, 142
Jonas Bronck Medical Center, xiv,
    10, 14, 35, 44, 45, 54, 55, 57, 59,
    61, 62, 66, 114, 165, 183, 185, 227
Jones, Erica, 123–24, 127
Joubert syndrome, 79

Kawasaki disease, 160–61, 162, 163

lab technicians, 69–72
power of, 65–66
Lederman, Dr. Delia, 168–71, 173

leukemia, 78
Lindsay, Dr. Scott, xiii, xiv, 2, 6–7,
    78–79, 103–4, 107–8, 150–52,
    154–55, 218, 234–37, 244–45,
    250, 251, 255
coping mechanisms of, 180–82
and "doctor's orders war," 74,
    76, 77, 79–85
effects of internship on, 27, 251
first on-call experience of, 25–28,
    103–4
problems with nurses, 74, 75–76,
    80, 82–83, 152, 245
relationship with girlfriend, 7
loculated pneumonia, 61
Logan, Dr. Ned, 84–85, 126, 127
lymphadenopathy, 109

managed care, effects of on
    delivery of care, viii–x, 89
Marion, Beth (wife), 2, 10–14, 23,
    24–25, 36, 100–101, 102, 103,
Marion, Dr. Robert, 2–6, 23–25, 28,
    35–45, 65–74, 81–82, 84, 87–89,
    100–103, 109–12, 131–41,
    159–63, 210–14, 231–34, 246–48,
    251–54
fears of, 3, 231–32
first on-call experience of, 23–24
post-call experience of, 100–101,
    103
problems moving to Boston, 2–3,
    36
problems with attending
    physicians, 43–44
problems with lab technicians,
    69–74
Match Day, 16, 196, 200–201, 204
procedure for, 197–98
Memorial Sloan Kettering
    Hospital, 32, 154
Miller, Dr. Mike, 155, 172, 185, 186,
    187

Morgan, Dr. Neal, 160–61, 162
Mount Scopus Medical Center, xiv,
    7, 29, 45, 76–77, 84, 107, 122,
    154, 202, 216
Murphy, Dr. Donald, 132–33, 164

Nathan, Dr. Julie, 10, 11, 14. *See also*
    Goodman, Dr. Andrea
National Residency Match, 149
New England Journal of Medicine,
    111, 129
neurofibromatosis, vii–viii, ix
New York Hospital, 144
Nieves, Caroline, 121–22, 129
non-Hodgkins lymphoma, 29–33
nurse practitioners, 55, 62–63, 259
    attitudes of interns toward, 55,
        62–64
nurses, 57, 77, 181
    attitude of interns toward, 78, 80,
        188–89, 190–91, 216, 260
    problems with interns, 75–76,
        80–81, 82–85

omphalocele, 233–34
orders, writing up of, 77–78
osteogenic sarcoma, 79

pancytopenia, 114
Park, Angela, 28–33
physician's assistants, 62
    attitude of interns toward, 55,
        62–64
Pneumosystis carynii pneumonia,
    112, 114–15, 118, 120
polycystic kidney disease, 14
Powers, Dr. Denise, xiii, xiv, 2, 7–8,
    92–93, 114–17, 122, 152–54,
    215–19, 251
    attitude toward nurse
        practitioners and physician's
        assistants, 55, 62–63
    car problems of, 7–8, 53

coping mechanisms of, 64, 182
    effects of internship on, 217–18,
        251
    problems with attending doctors,
        53–60
    stress of moving to Bronx and,
        7–8
pulmonary sequestration, 61

Reid, Dr. J. Cuthbert, 46–51
    and treatment of housestaff, 47,
        49–51
Richards, Dr. Jim, 15
Richardson, Molly, vii–x
Rivers, Randy, 110–11

St. Ann's Hospital, 4, 17, 23, 24, 25,
    28, 37, 39, 43, 247
scrub suits, 93–95
Sherman, Dr. Jesse, 175
Silverberg, Dr. Herb, 59–60, 61–62
Smith, Monica, 114–15, 116–17,
    129
Stark, Drs. Larry and Andrea,
    240–43

Tanner, Dr. Terry, 228, 230
Turner, Lucille, 228

University Hospital, xiv, 66
University of Pittsburgh, 17

Watson, Andre, 134–37, 138–40
Weinstein, Dr. Luise, 144, 145, 146
West Bronx Hospital, xiv, 74, 150,
    152, 153, 180, 187, 188, 194, 245,
    249–50
Winston, Dr. Matt, 65, 66, 109, 111

Zion, Libby, 144–45, 146. *See also*
    Weinstein, Dr. Luise
Zion, Sidney, 146–47, 149, 255. *See
    also* Bell Commission